PASSING THROUGH THE STORM

PRAISE FOR DENNIS SNODGRASS

I have had the honor to work with Dennis for several years. In that time, Dennis partook in training several groups around the United States. His personal story and connection to distracted driving had a substantial impact on the safety culture of our organization. His story helped us achieve the next level in vehicle safety both on and off the job. Thank you, Dennis!

— R. KELLY GEORGE, VICE PRESIDENT
ENVIRONMENTAL, HEALTH AND SAFETY RAIN
FOR RENT (MENTOR AND FRIEND)

———

In 2005, while deployed with the Army in Balad, Iraq, I read an article about a young woman who suddenly died in a car accident while leaving her fiancé's funeral. The tragedy of that story struck a cord and stayed with me over the years, often coming to mind throughout my career.

Eight years later, I found myself in Minot, ND starting a new career, sitting through a safety class on distracted driving. Imagine my surprise when our safety manager, Dennis Snodgrass, told the story of how his sister was tragically taken in a car accident caused by distracted driving, while leaving her fiancé's funeral. The jolt of realization as the article I read nearly a decade ago sprang to the forefront of my mind, that Dennis' sister was the young woman whose story had haunted me through the years left me reeling.

The impact of Dennis's story, his personal tie, and the passion of his presentation has had a lasting effect on how I drive and has surely saved countless lives. Dennis has devoted his career to telling his sister's story in hopes of changing driving habits and increasing awareness of the dangers of distracted driving.

— JOHN "GUS" VOGT

PASSING THROUGH THE STORM

DENNIS SNODGRASS

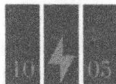

For my Family

CONTENTS

"Life is 10% what happens to us and 90% how we react to it."

— Dennis P. Kimbro

INTRODUCTION

My hotel window framed the stunning Houston skyline. The buildings were gently lit by the early morning sunrise. I scanned the parking lot packed with vehicles coated in a light dew that had accumulated the previous evening. The leaves on a small tree waved in a tender breeze, wishing me a good morning. I was no stranger to Houston. In fact, I had been here a couple times and knew full well that in a few short hours, this quiet and peaceful beauty would be transformed into a fast-paced business metropolis forced to endure the intense heat the local news channel forecasted.

Over the years, I'd grown used to traveling from city to city and living in random hotels. On these work trips, I typically found myself waking up to the gentle ring of my cellphone. Mitzie, the love of my life, got me off to a good start and wished me a wonderful day. Today, that wouldn't be necessary. For whatever reason, I woke early and decided to call to wish her well.

My half-filled cardboard cup held barely warm coffee. I took a deep breath, nursed my drink, and I continued to stare out at the wide swath of lights. I was mentally preparing myself for what was sure to be a very busy day. I had delivered this presentation countless times, and I found myself thinking back to the event that eventually became the inspiration for my lecture. I took another sip and allowed my thoughts to drift back and settle on the untimely death of my youngest sister, Michelle.

My older sister Penny had called to tell me about Michelle's car accident. Although it had happened several years earlier, the sting was just as strong. I'll never forget that call as long as I live.

"I think we've lost her." Penny's broken voice delivered the haunting message.

Her words crackled through the phone that chilly October evening.

"What do you mean we lost her?" I asked.

Thoughts were running through my mind like an auctioneer belting out a rhythmic series of bids, but the pounding from deep inside my heart told me that this wasn't good. Maybe it was the fateful words my sister chose to use. Maybe it was her tone. I just sat there in un-wanting anticipation, waiting for the bad news.

The event forever changed the lives of all my family members. My little sister, Michelle, died in an automobile accident on a rain-soaked highway near the coast of North Carolina. She was only thirty-two years old, and her life was over. Her life may have ended in that accident, but her story certainly didn't.

1

THE EARLY YEARS

Michelle's life began in the sleepy Northwestern Pennsylvania town of Coudersport. On Friday, June 1, 1973, at Charles Cole Memorial Hospital, our parents, John and Gail, welcomed the last of their six children into the world. They named her Michelle Lea. She was born with a head full of curly, coal-black hair. Michelle had three brothers. I was the eldest brother at five years old, followed by our brother Mike. While he was growing, Mike was a curious child. He was that kid who would take things apart and intently study each component, trying to figure out how it functioned. Later in life, he developed an interest in music, and eventually he became a very talented drummer. Chris, a couple years younger than me, was adopted by our aunt and uncle when he was a small child. He always felt like a cousin to us. I don't remember him ever living in our home. Along with her brothers, Michelle had two sisters, Penny and Denise. Being older than the rest of us, Penny seemed to be so much wiser than we were. It was almost as if she was an adult in our eyes. Denise was always the loudest of all of us kids. I think Michelle may have gotten some of her personality from Denise. Denise wasn't afraid of anyone and would fight at the drop of a hat. If someone pushed her too far, she was quick to meet the challenge. We also had a half-sister, Sherry, who came from our father's earlier relationship.

When Michelle was born, we lived in Shinglehouse, Pennsylvania, approximately twenty miles from Coudersport. Shinglehouse is a small village nestled in a hilly valley in Potter County with approximately two thousand residents. Many of the residents were relatives from our mother's side of the family. Many more that weren't related to us may as well have been. They were as close to us as our family was. There wasn't much employment in Shinglehouse at that time. The town consisted of a grade school, high school, a couple of gas stations, a hardware store, a rundown lumber mill, some local bars which were more like local gossip joints, a fire department, and Shorty's bicycle shop.

Our family was relatively poor. Our father struggled to keep a running vehicle on the road to shuttle us around for groceries, activities, and to visit our relatives. Most visits were to our grandmother, Edna, and Smokey, her live-in mate we considered our grandfather. As children, we loved going to Gram and Smokey's home. Smokey always had kind words for the grandchildren, and he would sneak us various snacks of mostly candy. Our grandmother was a kind lady whose favorite pastime was going to bingo at the area fire departments. She knew every bingo hall all over northern Pennsylvania, and they all knew her. My favorite memories include Gram's cooking. It seemed as though every dish she prepared was a delectable treat. She was a huge influence on our mother. Not only could mom prepare delicious meals like her mother, but she also loved to periodically make the bingo circuit with Gram.

At times, our father spent years in between jobs. Some of this was due to a depressed local job market and living in a small, remote town with very little to offer. He could have also lacked motivation because another portion of his unemployment history was due to an unfortunate disability. When our father was a teenager residing in rural West Virginia, he suffered severe burns to his right hand and lower arm while smoking near an open gas can. This injury left him badly scarred and barely able to bend most of his fingers. In fact, he couldn't move two of his fingers at all. To this day, I firmly believe this injury scarred more than just his right hand. I also think it had a lifelong impact on his confidence, mainly due to the limited ability that he had to effectively use that hand.

Throughout our younger years, we moved around quite a bit. We never stayed in one place for too long. Hell, we were a lot like nomads. Our parents had a gypsy heart with a lifestyle to match, and they weren't afraid to uproot their family and move on whenever they felt the time was right. Good, bad, or indifferent, I believe all of us kids inherited this trait from them. In time, we each demonstrated our free spirits, and we lived in separate states. Frequently moving around had a significant impact on our ability to make and retain friends. This was difficult on us; however, it taught us how to adjust on the fly. We each became experts in adapting.

Michelle seemed to be the favorite child. In time, I would learn that this isn't all that uncommon for the youngest child, but somebody failed to let the rest of us kids in on that fact. We were always a bit jealous and somewhat bitter. It was mainly because our treatment was anything but equal. Mom was a sweet woman with a big heart. Her biggest fault was that she would allow people to take advantage of her kindness. Our father was a strict disciplinarian and had no qualms with harshly disciplining his children. We would often find ourselves on the business end of a leather belt or a hand-picked switch from a nearby tree when we would misbehave. At times, he would whip us until he got tired. In his younger years, he seemed to have a great deal of stamina. Mom much disliked the way Dad disciplined us kids; it would often lead to some very loud arguments. We all knew when our father was upset. As a result, we would walk on eggshells when we were around him. But Michelle never seemed to have this problem. In fact, Dad would usually baby her while holding the rest of us accountable. Sometimes, we were in trouble for stuff she would do. We all had to be very careful when we would pick on Michelle for fear that she would run to Dad and tattle on us. It didn't take her long to figure out her preferential status and use his selective treatment to her advantage. She always seemed to have a sneaky side to her and a rather devious giggle as well.

We all got used to our youngest sibling's easier path, and we came to accept it. There wasn't much we could do about it. Even though growing up was a little less stressful for Michelle, she wasn't weak. All things being equal, Michelle may have been the strongest-willed child of all of us, and she was physically strong as well. She was as tough as nails. She never seemed to care what people thought of her, and later on in life, she would be more than willing to voice her opinion to whoever she felt needed to hear it. She openly displayed her strength early on. As a small child, Michelle nearly destroyed her baby crib, earning her a nickname, "Tiger." She really enjoyed this nickname. Throughout her life, it was common to see tigers in all forms with her. From stuffed animals to small ornaments and keychains; she proudly displayed her well-earned epithet.

———

A FEW YEARS AFTER MICHELLE'S ARRIVAL, OUR FAMILY relocated to Mannington, West Virginia, establishing a residence on Marshall Street. This would be the first of many new addresses. In fact, we would move so much while growing up, it eventually stopped surprising us when it happened. We would simply sit back and wonder when it was coming. Mom and Dad settled us into a large Victorian home in a relatively quiet neighborhood. Mannington was Dad's childhood home, and

Marshall Street was a couple blocks away from the school where he graduated. His former high school was converted into a grade school where my siblings and I attended, at least for a little while. It was also somewhat close to a city park and a little shop that sold ice cream and pepperoni rolls, which many locals considered a true West Virginia delicacy.

Mannington was a fun town, even though we never really ventured too far away from our house. It was much bigger than Shinglehouse, so we kept our exploring to within a three or four-block radius. We were all used to living in a small town. In Shinglehouse, we could ride our bikes from one end to the other in roughly twenty minutes, and nearly everyone who saw us, knew who we were or who we belonged to. But hardly anybody knew us in Mannington. We were just the new kids in town, and we would often get bullied or picked on by the local children.

After some time, we started making friends in our little neighborhood. We each also quickly settled in to our individual routines. Michelle was much smaller than the rest of us and primarily wanted to tag along with her sisters every chance she got. It was hard to ignore her, and she had a knack for standing out in a crowd. Maybe it was because she tended to be rather loud, or maybe it was because she was very independent.

It wasn't long before Michelle's independent spirit would be on full display and at a bit of embarrassment to our parents. One day, Michelle was given a small bag of used clothes that were donated at her pre-school. While on the bus ride home, she decided she wanted to try on some of her new clothes and proceeded to do just that. Off with the old, and on with the new. That was Michelle. With her, we expected the unexpected. If nothing else, she was rather entertaining.

She remained the apple of our father's eye, which we resented to a certain degree. But my brother, sisters, and I quickly became very protective of our baby sister, and we would often place ourselves in peril to make sure she didn't get hurt. As much as we didn't want to admit it, she would become the apple in each of our eyes as well. It was our job to look out for her, and she kept all of us on our toes.

Although we all made some pretty good memories in Mannington, we barely had enough time to get comfortable before we would relocate to another home in another town. With the exception of Penny, the rest of us were a bit too young to be largely impacted by this rather sudden move. It came as a result of our parents securing a job in a nearby town. We could have remained where we were, but they thought it would best to get closer to their place of employment. For me, Mannington turned out to be just a blip on the radar, and it ended in a blink of an eye.

Our new home was located a few miles down the road in the small mining town of Farmington. We settled into a small, one-story, ranch-style home on a hill overlooking the town. Farmington was a quiet country village that was more like we were all used to. There were not many businesses in this small town, and in order for most of the residents to be gainfully employed, a solid vehicle was a necessity. Although quaint and rather tucked away in the West Virginia wilderness, Farmington was mostly known for a tragic mining accident in the late sixties. A fire ignited in the depths of the Consol No. 9 Mine, taking the lives of many coal miners. Our new home sat directly above the infamous mine. The long, jagged cracks in the foundation walls and the large, deep caverns that surrounded our property reminded us of the shaky ground we lived on. We played around these holes, and it's a wonder none of us ever fell into any of them. Unlike Mannington, the school in Farmington was much smaller and seemed more inviting to us. We still found ourselves occasionally being picked on and ridiculed, mainly because we were poor and didn't have much. For the better part of the time, we were accepted by the locals. This was where Michelle began grade school.

The new neighborhood provided us kids with open fields to play in and room to roam, which was something that we didn't have a lot of in Mannington. Farmington was a small picturesque town that you might find displayed on a postcard in a wire rack exhibit at the local drugstore. Compared to Shinglehouse and Mannington, Farmington was the first place I finally felt at home. The house was quite small, and quarters were tight, but we made the best of it. Our older sister, Penny, grew to a young adult and gave birth to her first child, Jon. My brother Mike, my twin sister Denise, and I were bringing our elementary years to an end and looked forward to middle school. Aside from having to scale what seemed like a mountain on a daily basis, living on the hill was fun. We always found things to do. This hill provided some challenges on a daily basis, and we didn't realize just how dangerous it was navigating the winding paved roads that weaved their way up the side of this perceived mountain to our home.

It was on our hill that Mike and I taught Michelle how to ride a two-wheel bicycle. Standing at the top, we steadied the bike and helped her up on the seat. She could barely reach the peddles, and her arms were stretched straight as she gripped the handlebars. With one hardy shove, Michelle made her way down the steep hillside, complete with cracked and partially heaved pavement. Of course, we forgot to verify whether she knew how to apply the brakes. It was soon evident that she had no clue about brakes, and we had no clue what speeds she reached. While screaming down the hill, Michelle maintained her balance. About midway down, the seat loosened and fell off the bicycle, and our unsuspecting little sister sat down on the connecting tube. Although it clearly hurt her behind, she displayed her toughness and handled the hill very well, resulting in a huge sigh of relief from my brother and me. We certainly didn't want to explain to our father what happened, and to her credit, Michelle never complained about it.

We spent the majority of our free time hanging out with a

local family that lived a few houses down the street from us. The McKinney's were a family much like ours. They seemed to have a child in each of our age groups, which made making friends easy for everyone. I was especially smitten with the oldest girl, Melissa. I thought for sure that we would marry when we both grew up. When we weren't trying to together navigate the mountainous slopes on our mostly cobbled bicycles, we all played baseball, tag, or hide-and-seek in a large field that our parents had painstakingly mowed down for us. I thought that we were going to live there forever, and of all of my childhood homes, the one in Farmington harbors the fondest memories. Just as we began to think that we had finally become stable and found our forever home, Mom and Dad began discussing a potential move north.

———

IN 1980, OUR FAMILY RETURNED TO PENNSYLVANIA. Moving from place to place was an event that was becoming all too familiar at this point. This move was an unpopular one with us kids. We liked it where we were and had finally made some real friends. We had friends that didn't judge us for not having much. They accepted us for who we were and that meant a lot to us, so it was tough to say goodbye. Strangely, there seemed to be a bit of adventure to this move. Even as a child, I realized that leaving was simply a part of our lives, and I decided then that I would never allow myself to get too comfortable in one place ever again.

During this time, Penny was also going through a transition. She soon ventured out on her own to begin her life as an adult. She would eventually settle in the town of Genesee and then on to Wellsboro. We missed her and would often go long periods without seeing her. This was significant, because for everything we seemed to be lacking as children, we always had each other.

Now a member of the gang was gone. Sadly, this was something we all would have to get used to as well. When you are a part of a family that becomes as mobile as ours was, members of that family begin to venture out on their own, and schedules rarely match up. The winding roads of life tend to travel in much different directions. Penny and our parents were certainly moving in very different directions.

Moving back to Pennsylvania wasn't entirely bad. It put us closer to our favorite cousins, Ronda and Juny. They were more like good friends than cousins, and we all enjoyed hanging around with them. Ronda and Juny's mother, Aunt Rosie—who was lovingly referred to as "Little Rosie," because of how short she was—seemed to enjoy having us kids around and always treated us well. Their dad, Uncle Ronnie, made sure that we were included in some of their family events. The two of them would often go out of their way to make us feel part of their family. Ronnie and Rosie were almost like a second set of parents.

Mike and I spent the majority of time running around with Juny, while Denise and Ronda would go their own way. I was always impressed with Ronda and Juny because, unlike my siblings and me, they never missed a day of school. When we all began our high school years, Michelle was still a bit too little to hang out with Denise and Ronda, but she would always try to tag along and be everywhere they were. This wouldn't always be the case. Later in life, Michelle and Ronda would become very close. Even though there were a few years' difference between them, they would spend time with each other. Uncle Ronnie was always a huge baseball fan, and you could often find him in front of a television catching a game or two. Aunt Rosie was always working on some sort of craft, whether it was a cross-stitching project or crocheting something. She was very creative and always seemed to be happy. I always enjoyed our sleepovers because they would have snacks, especially pizza, before bed.

This was something that we didn't get a lot of at home, so I looked forward to these times.

In time, we would continue to move from town to town and state to state. Denise eventually left our home to join the Job Corps, and the rest of us moved away to the small town of Beverly, Ohio. Mike, Michelle, and I really liked Beverly, but when we first moved into the area, we lived a minimal existence for a while. We moved in to a rundown cabin that belonged to a family friend. It included a bedroom, kitchen and living room combination, and a bathroom with a shower. If we hadn't already developed survival skills, this cabin certainly aided in that process. Due to the number of people trying to exist in such a small space, this living arrangement would often test our patience. We also had the honor of experiencing something most kids our age never get the opportunity to. This cabin wasn't equipped with an indoor toilet. When we needed to do our business, we had to wander outside to an outhouse, regardless of the weather. Thankfully, the harsh living conditions didn't last very long. Mom eventually landed a job as a cook at a local restaurant, and we were soon able to move into a small, two-bedroom apartment a few blocks from the schools. It wasn't much, but compared to the rustic cabin, it was a mansion.

Living in the cabin shouldn't have been too difficult for Dad. He spent all of his younger years raised in a rustic log cabin outside Mannington, West Virginia, close to the small town of Metz. His childhood home was built by his father on a wooded hillside with a long and narrow road winding its way up from Route 250. To get there, you had to drive across a hand-built bridge that spanned Buffalo Creek and drive a rough mile and a half. Due to the immense canopy of trees, the road always seemed to be dark and desolate. It was chiseled out of the rocky hillside, complete with a steep drop-off to one side. I don't believe this manmade road had a legally recognized name, but years later the hill was often referred to as Snodgrass Mountain.

Dad talked to us kids quite often about his meager upbringing on the hill, and he would share details of what life was like in their log cabin. I didn't see the cabin up on top of that hill because my grandfather died before I was born and my grandmother had moved to Macksburg, Ohio shortly thereafter. All of my memories of the hill were from when we would visit with our cousins, Charlie, Dwight, and Beth. My Uncle Jack and Aunt Ethel homesteaded up there, and later on so did their boys.

While in high school, I had the opportunity to see the cabin that our father spoke so dearly of in his many stories. It was eventually disassembled and moved off the hill and reassembled on the opposite side of Route 250 on a neighbor's property. Dad took me over to look at it shortly after we moved to Ohio. There didn't seem to be much space in the small, box-shaped structure. I remember wondering how a large family could live comfortably in such a small home, but he always said that he enjoyed living there. At the time, I felt as though I was being taken back in time and introduced to a piece of my family's history.

I enjoyed going to school at Fort Frye High School in Beverly. This was probably the first place where we didn't become victims of bullying. The local kids didn't seem to mind that we were very poor, and we made many friends. In fact, we were quite popular among the locals. Much like in Farmington, Beverly felt very much like home to me. I played varsity football, and Michelle participated in the junior high school band. We made the best of living in Beverly. Mike and I mainly hung out at the local pool hall and became fairly good at shooting pool and playing nine ball. At times, we would make a little extra cash hustling some local kids out of their spending money.

I did quite well in school as well. I was able to maintain A's and B's, and I thoroughly enjoyed going to class every day. There was just something different about living in Ohio, and I enjoyed nearly every day of our time there. I wanted it to last forever, but eventually the school year would come to an end.

After I graduated from high school, I became the third sibling to head out into the world. Denise had eventually made her way back home and joined us in Beverly, but I still counted her time away in the Job Corps as her heading out into the world. I joined the United States Marine Corps and soon departed for Parris Island, South Carolina, to attend basic training. As for the rest of my family, they moved back to Pennsylvania. If I didn't know better, I would have thought my parents were fugitives from justice or in the Federal Witness Protection Program.

2

THE ADULT YEARS

After returning from the Job Corps and joining us in Ohio, Denise settled into her post-school routine. Much to everyone's surprise, when she left the Job Corps, she parted with much more than just an education. She became pregnant while she was a student there, and upon moving to Beverly, gave birth to her first child, Brandie. Being young and trying to raise a child on her own proved to be a challenge for my sister, but she made it work out. Mom and Dad adored Brandie and helped Denise get on her feet as much as they could. She experienced the struggles that often accompany a young, single mother. For Denise, it was tough being alone, but she wouldn't be alone for long.

Denise soon met and fell in love with her future husband, Paul; however, everyone referred to him as Junior. After growing up in rural Ohio, not far from the Beverly area, Junior enlisted in the military and became a member of the U.S. Navy. He was serving aboard the USS Iowa, based out of Norfolk, Virginia. Denise met Junior through her roommate, while visiting some mutual friends in Waterford, Ohio. They seemed to hit it off almost immediately, and it wasn't long before they saw each other on a fairly regular basis. After dating for a while, their relationship became more serious. In 1987, Junior asked Denise to marry him, and she gladly said, "Yes." Although he wasn't Brandie's natural father, he accepted Brandie and Denise as a package deal and welcomed that responsibility. It wasn't long before Denise and Brandie left the relative quiet of Southeastern Ohio to live the military life and all its hustle and bustle in the much busier city of Norfolk. The move was convenient for me, because I was stationed at Camp Lejeune, North Carolina. Although I didn't visit as much as I would have liked to, I was rather content knowing my twin sister lived just a few hours north of me. It also helped that my older sister, Penny, resided a few hours to the west, in Greensboro. It was after Denise and Junior married and left for Norfolk when Mom, Dad, Mike, and Michelle departed Ohio and moved to Kane, Pennsylvania.

———

SETTLING IN KANE SEEMED TO BE A GOOD MOVE FOR our parents. After all the moving around and the seemingly endless miles logged, it finally appeared that they had found the place where they would be most comfortable. The move proved to be good for their bank account as well. Dad was able to find a solid job that paid decent wages. He was employed at Kane Hardwood, a wood mill that made cabinet door panels. For what it's worth, he seemed to enjoy working there. Kane Hardwood was the premiere place for employment. In an area with few opportunities, Dad was fortunate to secure one of them. He ran a glue press which allowed him to work productively with his nearly crippled hand. It was a bit of therapy for him, because it also required a significant amount of coordination with his hands. Mom, who was always a fantastic cook and had worked in the restaurant industry previously, went to work for a small family-style restaurant in downtown Kane. Looking in from the outside, it was fairly obvious that our parents were able to live much better than I had ever remembered. Mom and Dad were able to afford a much nicer apartment, and they purchased a newer vehicle. For the first time, they also seemed quite happy, and that is what mattered most to me.

The two remaining kids, Mike and Michelle, also seemed to like living in Kane. Mike was finishing up high school and discovering his musical talents while Michelle was just entering her final years of school and discovering her wild side. Her ever-evolving independence was also taking shape. She had her own group of friends that she hung out with, and occasionally she would find herself in some mischief. She wasn't the typical high school student. Although very smart and able to earn good grades, Michelle made high school quite difficult on herself, and she made things rather difficult on our parents. If she didn't want to attend on any particular day, she simply wouldn't. On more than one occasion, I remember listening to our mother attempt to explain Michelle's perceived lack of enthusiasm. We couldn't figure out why she was acting out so much. Perhaps it was the constant packing up and moving all the time. Maybe it was the fact that she was always able to essentially do whatever she wanted to and whenever she wanted to. I personally believe it was a combination of both. Michelle seemed to be lost at times. For all of her good points, she definitely lacked accountability. Michelle would eventually drop out of school and set her sights elsewhere. The engrained gypsy spirit took hold and would lead her on many sordid adventures in the years to come.

At some point in 1988, Mom and Dad granted Michelle permission to move down to Norfolk to live with Denise and Junior. I think they were hoping that Denise would be able to control Michelle's somewhat wild side and become a positive role model for her. Michelle was maybe sixteen, and Norfolk was a new stomping ground and supplied a completely new set of friends. If Mom and Dad were hoping that this move would change Michelle's path, they were sadly mistaken. Being away from the nest, Michelle discovered a greater level of freedom. Partying and late nights would also become a part of Michelle's new life away from the relative control of our parents.

Considering the immense size of the military and the number of people from every corner of the United States that inundated the Norfolk Naval Station, groups of friends often crossed paths and blended with one another. This was especially true with Denise and Junior's clique. Weekend parties and cookouts were commonplace on many military installations, and they were no stranger to those. There were many sailors attending these parties that Denise and Junior would, at times, play host to. It was here that Michelle's life would take a rather significant turn. A young man from Michigan showed up at one of these events and caught Michelle's eye. His name was Wesley. Wes, as he was more commonly known, had mutual friends with Denise and Junior. He was a relatively large man, easily standing better than six foot and weighing over two hundred pounds. He seemed to be a bit shy with a relatively quiet demeanor. Standing alongside the five-and-a-half-foot Michelle, he appeared to be a giant that towered over her. Michelle was smitten.

As time went on, Michelle and Wes grew closer, and it was apparent that they were in the process of taking their relationship to an entirely new level. When Michelle turned seventeen, she asked our parents for permission to marry Wes. With a bit of hesitation and perhaps some apprehension, Mom and Dad eventually granted Michelle and Wes permission to marry. On a very warm and breezy summer day, Michelle and Wes married in a backyard ceremony, planned and arranged almost completely by Denise and her friends. It was quaint, but it was a very nice ceremony, and Michelle looked quite happy. Just as Denise had done before her, Michelle would experience life as a military dependent and all the trials and tribulations that accompany it.

In May 1989, I also married. Shortly thereafter, my wife Rose and I welcomed the first of our two children, Amanda, into the world. A couple years later, we would have our second, a son we named Shawn after my best friend in the Marine Corps. Our brother Mike would also eventually marry and have two children of his own, Shaina and Cameron.

Michelle and Wes didn't waste much time in starting their family either. Not long after marrying, they brought the first of three sons into the world. They named him Andrew. With Andy at their side, Michelle and Wes lived in a small apartment outside the Naval base, not far from Denise. Getting used to marriage and motherhood presented many challenges for Michelle, but at least she had her sister Denise relatively close to her. In the military, things tend to move quite fast, and Michelle would soon learn how quickly things can change and everyday routines and lives can be disrupted. As with most military members, getting orders and having to change addresses would eventually follow. It did not feel odd or unusual to Michelle, but the move to their new duty station in New Jersey would be stressful. With Wes and little Andrew, she now had more than just herself to worry about.

Wes and Michelle would spend a couple years in New Jersey and would eventually add their second child, Jerry, to their growing family. With all of its many stresses and challenging moments, the United States Navy provided a great deal of security for military families, but this would be the final duty station for Wes. The military wouldn't be his lifelong career choice. Once he honored his military commitment, he and Michelle decided to leave the military life and New Jersey behind them. This came as a bit of relief for Michelle. She was never very comfortable living in New Jersey and was looking forward to moving on.

———

FRESH OUT OF THE NAVY, WES BEGAN TRANSITIONING

back to civilian life and moved Michelle, Andy, and Jerry back to his home state of Michigan. They would live in a couple places, but they spent the majority of time living in the city of Jackson, approximately forty-five minutes west of Ann Arbor. Michelle spent most of her time as a stay-at-home mother and occasionally worked a part-time job at a local grocery store. Wes continued being the bread winner of the family and secured employment as a guard at a local prison. Not too long after arriving in Michigan, Michelle became pregnant once again and soon gave birth to their third child, Benjamin.

My parents and I visited Michelle in Michigan a couple of times. In the beginning, she seemed to enjoy her life there and spoke favorably about it, but over time, I remember thinking to myself that she didn't appear to be content and didn't sound very happy when I would talk with her over the phone. A couple of years later, Michelle confided in Mom that her marriage was on the rocks and that Wes was becoming more controlling of her time. Soon, stories began to surface about physical abuse. I knew that at some point, our little sister would need to get out of this situation and may have to leave Michigan in order to do this. I openly encouraged this change. Up to this point, I had considered Wes a friend and welcomed him to the family, but if the abuse allegations were true—and I had no reason to doubt my sister—I would have no more time for him.

———

AFTER LEAVING WES, MICHELLE LOADED UP HER THREE children and moved to our parents' place in Caldwell, Ohio. By this time, our parents' living arrangements had pretty much stabilized. Michelle was looking for a fresh start. Her time in Michigan had been incredibly stressful, and she simply wanted to be around her immediate family, specifically Mom and Dad. The breakup of her marriage had taken a toll on her emotionally, and she was glad it was over, or so she thought. Michelle had thought that she was a safe distance from Wes, but this would prove to be untrue. One day while Michelle was away from our parents' apartment, there was a tap on Mom and Dad's door. Holding Benjamin in her arms, Mom opened the door to find Wes standing on the other side. He forced his way into the apartment. To this day, nobody knows how he found our parents' apartment —most notably, Michelle and her kids—, but he did. He was there to take them. Wes loaded two of their children up in his car, returned to Michigan, and immediately filed for sole custody. He was unable to take Andrew because he was with Dad visiting relatives in West Virginia. There was nothing Mom could do to prevent him from taking the children. Although Michelle physically had them in Ohio, she never established custody due to her financial situation, and Wes knew she wouldn't be able to contest him in Michigan. This event haunted Michelle for years to come.

By this time, Junior was also out of the Navy, and he, Denise, and their three children had moved back to Ohio, approximately a half hour away from Mom and Dad. Michelle would shuttle back and forth between our parents' residence and Denise's over the next year or so. She would work various jobs that often were accompanied by long hours and unpopular shifts. The wages were fairly low and not very rewarding, but she always seemed to make the best of each situation. No matter how bad things got or how tired she became, Michelle continued to try to find ways to get her children back. Michelle also had to learn to do something she had never had to do before, survive on her own.

As time marched forward, Michelle's divorce with Wes was eventually finalized, ending a very sad and bittersweet chapter in her life. Although she had family that she could trust to be there when she needed them, she knew that she would have to take care of herself, put herself together, and simply move on. Over time, Michelle could see that Andrew was missing his siblings, which ultimately placed her in an extremely tough position. As much as it hurt her, Michelle knew that Andrew needed to be with his brothers. She eventually gave up the battle and allowed him to move up to Michigan and join his brothers under their father's roof. With a crushed spirit, Michelle placed one foot in front of the other and simply moved forward with her life.

———

ALWAYS THE SOCIAL BUTTERFLY, MICHELLE BEGAN accepting employment in very public career fields, such as clerking at convenience stores or tending bar in small country dives littered throughout the area. Shortly after her divorce, she met and began a rapid courtship with a young man named John. I don't know if it was because she felt an overpowering need to convince herself that Wes had been firmly placed in her past or if John was a rebound relationship. Regardless of her reasoning, Michelle and John hastily married in a small wedding attended by very few guests. It was a short-lived marriage. So short, that many members of the family never had the opportunity to meet him. As quickly as he entered her life, he exited. Michelle, once again, found herself single, divorced, and alone.

Nearing her mid-twenties and twice divorced, Michelle was once again forced to pick up the pieces and move on with her somewhat shattered life. You could tell that not having her children with her was seriously affecting her, and she was paying some hefty tolls along life's highway. These were tolls that few could understand, and they would continue inflicting emotional pain for the remainder of her life. However, you rarely saw it on her face. She always seemed to have a stoic poker face and hardly showed any emotions.

Michelle continued to work and would occasionally revisit her wild side from time to time. Regardless of what she had going on in her personal life, she always found ways to keep herself busy and move forward. If nothing else, she maintained a positive outlook and found something good in nearly every situation. Michelle enjoyed meeting new people and hanging out with friends, which is why her choice in jobs seemed to suit her well. I think it was less about her wages and more about her place within the social fabric that gave her some importance. Having two failed marriages behind her, she remained alone, at least for a while, and devoted much of her free time to family and friends.

One evening, after finishing her shift at the bar, Michelle made her way over to Marianne's restaurant for a bite to eat. Marianne's was located off of Interstate 77 in Belle Valley. The restaurant was in an ideal location for travelers to rest and take in a hardy meal. The friendly eatery attracted diners and truckers from all over. It wasn't uncommon for Michelle to pop in from time to time and visit with her friends and enjoy a burger and a hefty plate of fries. She was fairly well-known by the other patrons and was often warmly greeted.

It was at Marianne's, during one of these late-night dinners, that Michelle met a friendly truck driver. Danny was much older than Michelle, nearly twenty years her senior, but that didn't seem to bother either of them. They struck up a conversation that would eventually become a close friendship. Through their periodic late-night talks, they realized that they had much in common. Both were divorced. Each had children. And they were both huge NASCAR fans. They really enjoyed each other's company and would continue to meet often. It wouldn't be long before Danny was making Belle Valley a regularly scheduled stop on his trucking route to take in a warm meal at Marianne's and visit with Michelle.

Soon their visits were becoming more and more frequent, and at some point, when she was entering her late twenties, they began officially dating each other. The arrangement was a bit troubling for our family. It wasn't necessarily their age difference. The biggest concern was wondering whether this was another rebound relationship or if it was sincere. Personally, I just wanted her to be happy, and she certainly seemed happy when she was with Danny. Of course, being as independent as she was, Michelle wasn't going to allow our concerns to change her mind. She was quite capable of making her own decisions and wasn't afraid to let you know, especially it if she thought you may be meddling in her business.

Danny didn't live too far from Michelle, so maintaining a relationship wasn't all that difficult. He lived a couple of hours south, near Charleston, West Virginia, in the suburb of St. Albans. When Danny wasn't traveling north and stopping in Belle Valley to see Michelle, she would make the somewhat short trip to St. Albans to be with him. Danny seemed to maintain her attention and calm her wild side down a bit.

I always liked Danny, and he was always a lot of fun to be around. By the time he and Michelle had gotten together, my marriage with Rose had ended, and I was living back in Ohio. My two children, Amanda and Shawn, lived with their mother in Pennsylvania, and I would drive back and forth to visit with them. When I wasn't with my children, I would occasionally accompany Michelle on her trips to West Virginia. Danny had what some would consider a warped sense of humor. That was something that I could easily relate to, because I too had a rather strange sense of humor. Danny also seemed to get along well with the rest of our family and always treated our parents with respect.

Sometime around 1997, Michelle and Danny decide that they wanted to get married. I always figured that this day would arrive, but I wasn't really prepared to once again hear the news. This would be Michelle's third swing at the bat, and so far, she had struck out each time. I was hoping, beyond all hope, that this would be the one. She seemed to be truly happy, and I thought they made a nice couple. An oddball couple, but nonetheless, a nice couple.

LIVING IN THE GREATER CHARLESTON AREA PROVIDED Michelle with many things to do and a seemingly endless supply of opportunities. Although she continued taking jobs with small stores and bars, she always set her sights higher and soon began taking college courses. She studied to become a phlebotomist, but she would never work in that career field.

After leading a single life for several years, I met Mitzie, who would eventually become my lifelong partner. She was a member of my Army reserve unit in Parkersburg, West Virginia. She almost immediately caught my eye. Much like me, she had two children, Zack and Jared, and was going through a divorce. We immediately connected and became good friends. Months later, when we began dating, I took her down to St. Albans to meet Michelle and Danny. Michelle and Mitzie got along well, and the four of us spent the weekend hanging out.

A couple months later, Mitzie and I learned that she was pregnant, and we would soon be welcoming another child into our family. Mitzie and I began discussing relocating to her childhood town of Minot, North Dakota. The job market in Southeastern Ohio was beginning to struggle, and Minot presented many more opportunities for us. Although it would be a significant distance from my parents and children, I wasn't afraid to move away from Ohio. I found myself looking forward to a new challenge in my life. Over the next few months, we meticulously planned our impending move out west.

During the following year, Mitzie and I made our long journey to Minot, North Dakota so she could be closer to her parents during her pregnancy. In August 1999, she gave birth to a baby boy that we named Nicholas. Michelle and Danny continued to reside in St. Albans until late 1999 or early 2000. The company that Danny worked for shut down their terminal and released their drivers. This came as a complete shock for Danny, because he was within a couple of years of qualifying for retirement. Danny had relatives that lived in South Carolina, so they decided that was where they were going to move to. Unsure of their future, he and Michelle packed up their belongings and headed south.

3

MICHELLE MEETS DEAN

After moving to South Carolina, Michelle and Danny got settled and began their new lives away from their familiar settings and friends in Charleston. Danny was able to secure another trucking job, and Michelle continued working in convenience stores. They moved in with Danny's uncle for a brief period, and with some help from Danny's relatives, they eventually transitioned into their own place. It appeared that they were easily adjusting to life in the south, at least on the surface.

Being much closer to Penny, Michelle would often travel up and visit with her. No matter where she was residing at the time, Michelle often made trips to visit with family. She could never be away for too long. She had a fondness for traveling, and she had no issues with driving long distances to see her brothers and sisters. She would always make time to go see Mom and Dad, no matter where they may be living at that particular time. Family was very important to Michelle, and she rarely allowed anything to interfere with her visits. It had been quite a while since Mitzie and I had seen her. Denise and Mom were the only ones, up to this point, that had come out to North Dakota and visited with us since we left Ohio. I knew that it would only be a matter of time before Michelle would find herself traversing the country to Minot.

We hadn't seen her since our last trip to Charleston. Each of our lives were becoming so busy that we would often go weeks without even talking on the phone. Mitzie and I had talked a couple times about taking a vacation to Myrtle Beach so we could visit with Michelle and Danny. They didn't live far from there, and the trip would also allow us to go to the beach. Of course, it was one thing planning something, but it was entirely different executing those plans. Minot was a long way from South Carolina, and it takes a considerable amount of resources to make a trip like that. Certainly, more than we could afford at that time.

As days turned into months, Michelle hinted that her marriage was beginning to sour. I'm not sure if it was because of their significant age difference or if there was something a bit deeper, but it certainly appeared that they were drifting apart. She seemed so happy in Charleston, so it was possible that living in South Carolina may have played a part in her unhappiness. When Danny would go out on the road for work, Michelle would find herself spending more and more time away from home, traveling up to North Carolina. As much as we all hated for Michelle to be unhappy, marriage number three was officially on the rocks.

As their marriage continued to fracture bit by bit, Michelle and Danny spent the majority of their time away from each other. While in North Carolina visiting with Penny, Michelle struck up a friendship with a young man named Dean. Like Danny, Dean was a truck driver. Of course, at that time, Michelle had no way of knowing just how far this friendship would go. She knew how the relationship would be viewed, especially by her family. One thing we all knew about Michelle was, she was an independent person, and she wasn't one to let something like a broken marriage get in her way. After all, they were only friends, at least for the time being. The last thing she wanted was another failed marriage, but her and Danny's differences were becoming too much to ignore.

Over the next few months, she tried to give her marriage another chance of survival, but it just wasn't meant to be. I believe Danny knew that she was giving her heart to another man, and he soon resigned himself to the fact that she would one day be gone. As things with Dean continued heating up, Michelle eventually moved to Wilmington, North Carolina to spend her time with him. She began working at a convenience store on Oleander Drive in Wilmington and devoted her free time riding shotgun in Dean's truck. This was something she was never able to do with Danny and never really showed an interest in previously. But things were much different with Dean. They were only a couple of years apart in age, and they seemed to spend nearly every waking moment with each other. Over time, Michelle slowly introduced Dean to the family and shared the news that she and Danny would soon be divorced.

I was a bit disheartened when I heard that Michelle and Danny were inching closer to a divorce. I really liked him and remembered some fun times we'd had during my visits in West Virginia. I was hoping that he and Michelle would make it, but this was between the two of them and they would have to get through it themselves. My first thought was that Michelle was once again going to be a divorced mother of three. I wasn't sure where she and Dean would end up, and I couldn't devote too much energy to worrying about it. All I was concerned with was her being happy, and I wished Danny well.

———

I REMEMBER THE FIRST TIME I SAW A PICTURE OF DEAN. He was a large, heavy man with a neatly trimmed beard and shoulder-length brown hair, parted down the middle. Mitzie and I hadn't yet met him in person, but we would soon get our chance. Denise's daughter Brandie and her young child, James, were staying with us at the time. Michelle and Dean were going to travel out with Denise to pick them up. Finally, Michelle was going to come and visit us in North Dakota. I was excited for her and Denise to come out and spend a little time with us, but mostly I wanted to visit with Michelle and make sure she was doing alright. I won't lie; I also wanted to make sure that Dean was a good man.

They arrived a couple days later, riding in a small van that was packed with clothes, blankets, and empty soda bottles. One by one, they stepped out of the van, displaying the look of exhausted travelers who had pushed through the night and stopped for nothing but food and fuel. I hadn't seen Michelle in a few years and found myself displaying a smile that stretched from ear to ear as she approached me.

"Hey Chelle," I said. Over the years, we abbreviated her name. I'm not sure why we did that but, she never seemed to mind. In fact, she would have probably answered to almost anything.

I reached out and pulled her close to me for a hug. I missed my little sister and was glad she finally made her way out to see us. I then directed my attention to Denise while Michelle embraced Mitzie. After giving Denise a huge hug, I turned and faced Dean. He was bigger than he had appeared in the pictures. As Michelle introduced him, he slowly reached out his hand to shake mine. With a soft southern drawl, he said, "Dean, nice to meet ya."

Shaking his hand, I returned the greeting, "Nice to meet you as well."

After exchanging pleasantries, we all made our way into the house so they could rest and we could sit down and visit. Denise immediately ventured into the bedroom that Brandie and James were using so she could give them hugs and kisses. It wasn't long before the three of them joined the rest of us in the living room for coffee and conversation. We all had much to catch up on, and I wanted to get to know Dean a little while they were there.

It was easy to see that Dean and Michelle cared a great deal for each other, but I had seen this before, and I was a bit skeptical. They sat close to each other on the sofa and held hands as they shared stories of their journey out to North Dakota. This was the first time Michelle had seen the northern plains and was quick to mention how boring the ride through North Dakota was compared to the wooded North Carolina scenery.

Something else that Michelle and Denise weren't used to seeing was a police cruiser sitting in the driveway. By this time, my career was in law enforcement. After starting off as a reserve deputy with the Sheriff's department, I was now the Police Chief for a three-man department in the small town of Velva. Growing up and even into my early adult years, I was almost always involved in a little mischief, so becoming a police officer wasn't exactly the career choice my family envisioned for me. This, of course, brought about a bit of joking between the two of them and some reminiscing of my younger and somewhat wilder days. I didn't mind that I was the butt of their jokes. They were having fun, and I really enjoyed sharing a few laughs with my sisters.

DEAN HAD MADE A WONDERFUL IMPRESSION ON ME. He was a genuinely kind person who appeared to be appreciative of everything he had in life. I was rather confident that he would take care of Michelle and they would make a good couple. With the exception of her pass-through marriage to John back in Ohio years earlier, I had witnessed her interactions with her ex-husbands, and I could tell that there was something very different with Dean. Thinking back, I never remembered her walking hand in hand with the others. It was almost as if she was a teenager who had just introduced everyone to her first boyfriend. She was definitely giddy and spent the majority of her time with a large smile on her face. It may have been a little wishful thinking on my part that she had finally found that one special person, that Mr. Right, to spend the rest of her life with. On the surface, the two of them seemed like they were well on their way to marital bliss. I was once again happy for her.

As much as Mitzie and I enjoyed everyone's company, we didn't get to visit for very long. Our time with them was far too short, and I was thrilled to have the chance to see each of them. Over the next few days, everything got back to normal. Michelle and Dean had made their way back to North Carolina, and Denise and Brandie had been safely delivered back to Caldwell, Ohio. Mitzie returned to her job with ING, and I resumed my duties with the police department.

I worked there for a couple years in Velva before accepting a chief position with the City of Mayville, approximately seventy miles north of Fargo. Although larger than Velva, Mayville was a quaint college town located four hours east of Minot, and it presented some new professional challenges for me. I had always wanted to work in a small college town police department, and Mayville provided me with that rather unique opportunity. Life seemed to be quite a bit different on the eastern side of North Dakota.

Before bringing Mitzie and the kids to Mayville, I was able to find a small, two story home for us to rent. It was close to the schools, and there was an older couple living next door that had a grandchild who was our son's age. Although there weren't a great deal of things to do in Mayville, it was a relatively short drive to larger cities near us. We had Fargo to the south and Grand Forks, a bit closer, to the north where we did the majority of our shopping. I settled into my new role with the department and began meeting people and getting more involved in the local community. Everything seemed to move much faster, however the job market wasn't as fruitful for Mitzie. After some time, she was able to find an administrative job with a struggling company that built grain trailer augers. She clearly wasn't happy being away from the familiar confines of Minot, but she was very supportive of me and made the best of it.

Our kids, Nicky and Jared, also became more comfortable with their new living arrangements. Zack was already out of high school and was attending college in Wyoming. He would eventually join us in Mayville before taking up a more permanent residence in Fargo.

As they grew older, the boys wanted a pet, so with the help of one of Zack's friends, we were able to get a Border Collie pup that we named Skeeter. For some odd reason, I felt the need to also provide her with a middle name. I'm not sure why, but it stuck with her. From the time we got her, she would forever be known as Skeeter Pete. She was a cute pup, and Nicky and Jared took to her almost immediately. We had tried to have pets in the past, but it always seemed as though the novelty wore off quickly and the kids soon lost interest. We would ultimately end up finding new homes for each of them. Before getting Skeeter, I explained to the boys that they would have to take an active role in caring for her if we were to keep this one. Of course, they both agreed. Nicky was so young that he really didn't care, he just wanted a puppy. After uprooting them and moving halfway across the state, I felt the need to make it up to the boys, which quickly helped me to cave to the idea of bringing in another pet. Besides, it didn't take Skeeter long to steal my heart with her big brown eyes, and I didn't mind having her around. She seemed to fit right in.

Over the next two years, I made a couple of trips out to Ohio to visit with Mom and Dad. It was always nice to be able to spend some time with them. It was also nice to be able to get my older children, Amanda and Shawn, for a few days. After leaving Ohio, I rarely got to see any of them and cherished the times when I could travel back home and visit. When Amanda and Shawn were younger, Mitzie and I would bring them out to Minot to spend the summers with us, but as they got older, their summer visits became less and less convenient. I don't think they liked the long hours on the road, and after a while, I stopped pushing the issue.

Once they were both old enough to start making decisions, I allowed them to decide whether they wanted to come out to our home.

One trip back to Ohio was especially memorable. I had spent nearly a week with Mom and Dad, and everything seemed to have gone well the entire time until I was getting ready to depart. Michelle happened to arrive earlier that day to spend some time with mom and dad, and something was different with dad. He seemed extra distant and quiet. He also had a lost and confused look on his face. I wasn't sure what was happening, and I was thinking that he was sad to see me leave. Over the next dozen hours or so, the vision of Dad continued to haunt me. I should have stayed until I knew he was alright.

On my way home, I stopped for the night in Des Moines. I called Mitzie to see how she was doing, and she told me about the events with dad that had transpired since I left. That gut feeling that had stuck with me all day had proven to be an instinct I should have acted on.

"Your dad's in the hospital," she said. I heard what she was saying, but something in her voice didn't sound right. "He had to have brain surgery today."

"You're kidding," I replied. I kept thinking that deep down inside I knew something wasn't right when I left. Feeling guilty for not stopping my vehicle when I noticed how he looked, my next thought was to immediately return to Ohio to be with him.

"I should go back," I told Mitzie. "I should be there."

"Michelle is with them. He's fine. The surgery went well, and he's awake and recovering," she said.

As usual, she was making complete sense. I was closer to Minot than I was to Caldwell, so turning around and driving back wouldn't make much sense. Besides, I was completely exhausted from the several hours on the road, and was looking forward to some sleep. I decided that I would call Mom or Michelle the next day to check on Dad.

"What happened to him?" I asked.

"He had an aneurism that was about to burst, so they did surgery on him. I guess it did rupture when they opened up his head," she responded. "Michelle got him back to the hospital just in time."

When I awoke the next morning, I called Mom and learned that Michelle had noticed Dad's odd behavior, like I did as I was leaving. She took dad to the doctor, where they ran a series of tests and scans on him. After getting him home, the doctor called a short time later to have him return to the hospital because they had noticed the aneurism and emergency surgery was needed. As bad as I felt for not stopping when I sensed something wasn't right with him, I was very happy that Michelle was there. With her quick thinking, she essentially saved Dad's life. He was going to be okay, and our family was very thankful to still have him with us.

It was at that moment that I realized just how close I had come to losing a parent. With the exception of grandparents and a couple of uncles, we hadn't really experienced losing close family members. When we were all very young, we had a cousin die from smoke inhalation in a house fire, but we were all a little too young to fully understand the gravity of the situation. Learning that dad was in the hospital and had just gone through brain surgery, brought to light just how quickly life can change and tragedy can strike. I don't know if a person can really ever prepare themselves for losing an immediate family member. I knew that I wasn't ready to lose any of mine.

Back in Mayville, Mitzie and I planned a trip for the following summer to Ohio and North Carolina. We made plans to visit with mom and dad for a couple of days, pick up Amanda and Shawn, and then drive to the beach to camp with Penny and her husband, Ed. They knew of a nice camping area near Wilmington called Fort Fisher. This would also give us the opportunity to see Michelle and Dean, because they only lived a few miles from there. This would be the first real vacation that Mitzie and I had taken together in quite some time, and I was really looking forward to it.

———

THE WEATHER IN OHIO WAS VERY PLEASANT FOR EARLY July. After living in North Dakota for the previous six years or so, I had forgotten just how nice it was to have a large canopy of trees above us to provide an abundance of shade. The northern plains certainly lacked in trees, but it made up for it with its vast openness and immense beauty. Mitzie and I sat on a blanket by the banks of Wolf Run Lake, outside Caldwell. The kids played along the shoreline, and Skeeter Pete was jumping in and out of the water fetching the occasionally tossed stick. We visited mom and dad for a couple of days, and then we headed down to Spring Lake, North Carolina to Penny and Ed's home. Mitzie and I had each taken two weeks off work in order to enjoy the prolonged family vacation.

It took us approximately eight hours to travel to Spring Lake; compared to the drive from North Dakota, it seemed like a trip to the grocery store. The heat in the Carolinas was much different than that in North Dakota and Ohio, and none of us were used to it, especially Skeeter. The plan was to leave her with Penny's son, Chris. Skeeter had never been away from us till now, but Penny and Ed had a dog of their own, so Skeeter would have a friend to play with. My biggest fear was that she would discover a poisonous snake or something else that we didn't have to worry about in Mayville.

After resting for the night, we followed Ed and Penny a couple hours down the road to Fort Fisher. The campground was beautiful, and the ocean was a short walk from where we set up camp. I had gone camping many times in the past, but I had never camped at the beach. I found it to be incredible and planned to make the most out of it. Mitzie and Penny took some time to go souvenir shopping on the strip near the campground while I ventured to the beach with the kids. Later that day, we watched some local kids catch small sharks off a pier that extended over an inlet. There was so much to do, but it was just as much fun feeding bread scraps to the raccoons. Oddly, I never really felt nervous about sleeping in a tent, even though there were several signs warning of alligators in the vicinity.

Michelle had to work the day we arrived. We didn't get to visit with her and Dean until the next day. Around dinner time, they arrived at the campground, and Michelle immediately began to play with the kids. Amanda seemed to remember her most, so she hung close to her, which prompted Michelle to invite Amanda to spend the night at her and Dean's place. After we ate, we sat around and shared stories about times past. It wasn't long before Dean began to look as though he wasn't feeling well. I remember thinking that it was probably a touch of the flu or something. Michelle mentioned that they probably wouldn't be staying long, but they would be back the next day to return Amanda and continue visiting.

After Michelle and Dean had left, we began the process of settling the kids in for the evening and spending some quality visiting time with Penny and Ed. The coast was incredibly beautiful when the sun went down. I couldn't get over just how loud the ocean was when everything else becomes quiet. It took me back to my time in the Marine Corps, just an hour or so north of Wilmington. My friends and I would spend countless hours hanging out at the beach. Mitzie made us all some much-needed coffee, while the kids enjoyed a snack before heading off to bed. The beautiful roar of the ocean was occasionally broken by sounds of laughter from nearby campers having some fun and enjoying a few beers.

Mitzie and I wished everyone a good night and took ourselves to bed. I couldn't wait till morning to head back to the beach with the kids and spend a couple hours swimming. Although our air mattress was comfortable, I was unable to sleep because the air in the tent was very warm. Not having an air conditioner is probably the biggest disadvantage to camping in a tent. After a couple hours of laying on top of the blankets, I was finally able to get comfortable enough to drift off to sleep.

The next morning, I awoke to the sound of Mitzie's voice letting me know that breakfast was nearly done. The inside of the tent was extremely bright and the hot Carolina sun was already delivering a relentlessly powerful blast of heat. I felt as though I had spent the night in an oven. My skin glistened with a copious amount of sweat. It was as if I had just finished a short morning jog. Dragging myself out of bed, I rubbed the sleep out of my eyes and shuffled my way outside to enjoy some morning coffee.

Shortly after finishing breakfast and cleaning up, Michelle and Dean arrived with Amanda. Dean still didn't appear to be feeling very well. He was quieter than I had remembered and seemed to be somewhat withdrawn as we talked. I didn't know what was wrong with him, but I had a feeling it was something more than just the flu. Regardless of how bad he was feeling, they stayed for the better part of the day to spend some time with us. As the sun began to set, they departed for the night and we all prepared to bring another wonderful evening to a close.

Michelle came alone out to the campground the following day to see us off. Dean still wasn't feeling well. This was odd for them. They were always together. It was a brief visit and was mainly spent exchanging hugs and well wishes. Michelle seemed to be in a jovial mood, and she periodically belted out her signature laugh as she chased the kids around in an effort to plant a series of kisses on their cheeks.

"Tell Dean to get feeling better," I told her.

"I will big brother. Y'all have a safe trip back," she responded.

After delivering her hugs and kisses to the kids, she opened her car door, and continued waiving her hand as she climbed back into the driver's seat. With one hand in my pocket, I raised the other and waived back to her and watched her slowly pull away.

"I can't wait to see you again," I thought to myself, as I watched her taillights fade away in a cloud of dust kicked up by her tires. The dust dissipated, and I felt time steal the moment from me as I went back to the normality of life.

4

DEAN'S ILLNESS AND DEATH

After arriving home from North Carolina, Michelle called to have one of our periodic chats. However, this time I sensed that something wasn't right. I could tell that she had something weighing on her mind. I didn't want to pry, but I felt the need to ask her if there was anything she wanted to talk about.

"What's up Chelle?" I asked. "Everything all right?"

She didn't answer right away. It was almost as if she was contemplating how to put the words together. "Dean's got cancer," she responded. The urge to break down and cry was evident in her trembling voice. I could hear the wound; she was incredibly hurt.

I remembered our time down at Fort Fisher and how uncomfortable Dean appeared while we were all visiting with each other. I recalled how he looked unwell and thought it was a common cold or the flu. I never thought that he was suffering with this dreaded disease.

He's so young, I thought to myself.

I couldn't imagine what they were going through. The emotions and the pain that he was almost certainly experiencing must have been dreadful. More disconcerting was the uncertainty that the future held for both of them. I felt so bad for Dean. I don't know what I would do if I was in a similar situation. I'm not sure what I would say if I ever had the opportunity to even talk with him. He was a great guy, and things like this should never happen to anyone, especially great people like Dean. As bad as I felt for him, my heart broke for my sister. Michelle had never gone through anything like this before, and I'm sure she didn't even know how to handle this terrible news that they had been given.

I had so many questions that I wanted to ask her, but I really didn't know where to start. I really wished that I was right there with her. Sensing that she was about to cry, I simply uttered, "Are you okay?"

"About as good as I can be, I guess." Her voice was distant, and she just sounded lost. It was hard for me to fathom what was going through her mind or just how helpless she must have been feeling. I couldn't ever remember hearing her sound so vulnerable. She was always a strong woman, but with all of her experiences, life had toughened her up. Regardless of all the tough times that she had previously gone through, nothing could have prepared her for this. It was hard for all of us to hear of Dean's cancer diagnosis, but Michelle would have to personally deal with this disease and the terrible effects that it would have on Dean.

I maintained the belief that the doctors would find a way to cure him of this disease. After all, you hear stories all the time about people who have been diagnosed with cancer, and after some chemotherapy treatments, they go from cancer patient to cancer survivor. Dean's form of cancer was non-Hodgkin's lymphoma, which affects the lymphatic system. I've learned through some research that this is a fairly common form of cancer. So surely, he would be able to beat it. We all prayed and hoped, and Michelle continued to describe his various setbacks and daily struggles. But it wasn't long before I realized that his condition wasn't getting any better. This was still very unreal to me. He always seemed to be so big and strong, and I couldn't get the thought out of my mind of how young he was. As sad as I felt for Dean, I couldn't imagine how his family was doing. They had to be a wreck.

Dean's condition worsened, and it caused him to become increasingly less active. One of his and Michelle's favorite places to go was to the beach. I don't blame them. I have always found something incredibly therapeutic about walking on the warm sand and listening to the beautiful rhythmic music of the ocean. If anything, a trip to the beach would help Dean feel a little better.

One beautiful sunny day, Wrightsville Beach called to Penny, Michelle, and Dean. It would be great to enjoy some sand, surf, and sun. Michelle wanted to gather some seashells, and so they planned a walk, but Dean wasn't feeling up to it. He encouraged them to go on without him and sent them on their way.

On the beach, Penny talked with Michelle about Dean's illness. She wanted to make sure Michelle was okay. "Michelle, he doesn't look very good," Penny said. "You need to start preparing yourself."

"I know," Michelle responded.

Having Penny there with her helped give Michelle some much-needed strength. At least she wasn't having to go through this alone. We were all pretty much available anytime by phone, but Penny only lived a couple hours away, and that gave Michelle some comfort.

I didn't bother her much during this time. I knew that she had her hands full with shuttling Dean back and forth to his doctor's appointments and whatnot, but they were always on my mind. Her coworkers said that she always kept a smile on her face in front of them and the customers. But inside she was silently falling apart. She had been through so much; so much hurt, and so much pain. After three failed marriages, she was finally able to find her Prince Charming, and this terrible disease was going to take him away from her.

Once his condition deteriorated to the point he could no longer be at home, he was finally admitted to the hospital. Michelle, Penny, Ed, and Dean's family all camped out at the New Hanover Regional Medical Center and maintained a watch over him. They each took turns going into his room to quietly visit with him. He drifted in and out of consciousness, and Penny could tell that he was losing his brave fight.

The hands on the clock coldly and continually ticked on. Dean's parents left to get some rest, and the others promised to keep them informed of any changes in his condition. Soon a priest approached them. They collectively understood. The priest led them all back to Dean's room so each of them could quietly say their goodbyes.

A few minutes later, Penny went to the waiting room to take a breath and noticed Michelle hurriedly heading toward the door. Penny followed until she could see Michelle throwing up just outside. Dean had lost his brief fight and had gone home.

5

OCTOBER 6TH, 2005

Tropical storms aren't all that uncommon in the fall, especially this close to the coast. This October was no different, and a storm made its way up the coastline from Florida to Virginia, dropping considerable amounts of rain as it rolled along. There's never a good time for a tropical storm, but this one had incredibly bad timing.

The rain continued to pound the lush, dark green turf, creating small streams and channels that seemingly rolled on forever. The sun was elusive and nowhere to be found. The sky was normally lightly clouded with a splash of Carolina blue during the late fall days, but on this day, the sky was as dark and gray as freshly poured concrete. Weather like this typically forces residents to remain indoors, but on this day, a small funeral canopy attempted to shelter family, friends, and close acquaintances of big Dean. They came together to celebrate the beautiful life and an equally beautiful man. All were welcomed with the exception of one guest that invited herself to this somber gathering. Her name was Tropical Storm Tammy.

Funerals are difficult enough, but toss in a near-hurricane and it adds a completely new level of difficulty to the proceedings.

When the formal matters had wrapped up, the guests said their goodbyes, while a few were standing by to deliver hugs to whoever may have needed them. Many of the guests were going to journey to a dinner at Dean's parents' home. While speaking with Penny, Michelle mentioned that she needed to go to Andrew's Mortuary and then on to the convenience mart where she was employed, to purchase some cigarettes and a soda. "I'll be there in a few," she told Penny.

The drive was difficult to the dinner. Everyone that knew Dean had wrestled with their own sorrow and shock over his struggle and death. The storm reflected everybody's inner storms and made the drive exceptionally challenging. They each managed the journey and shortly after arriving at Dean's parent's place, Penny received a phone call from our mother. It didn't come as much of a surprise to get the call. She had been expecting her to check in on how the events had gone all day, but the rapid pace of Mom's voice and her sharp tone was disconcerting.

"I was just on the phone with Michelle, and I heard her say, 'Oh No,'" mom said. She sounded like she was holding back tears; the fear and panic were evident. "And the phone went dead!" she continued.

Penny assured mom that she would check around and attempt to find out what may have happened with Michelle. Because of the ferociousness of the storm, Penny reached out to the Highway Patrol to inquire about any vehicle accidents that may have recently happened. If Michelle was broken down or if her car was in some way disabled, somebody needed to get to her.

"Yes, we have a report of one on Highway 421, out by the USS North Carolina, but we don't have any further information," uttered the voice on the other end of the line.

With a tightness in her belly and thoughts racing through her mind, Penny knew she needed to go and see this accident scene for herself. Dean's aunt and uncle loaded Penny up, and together, they made their way to 421.

The red, flashing lights of fire trucks, ambulances, and police cars reflected off the waterlogged highway. Still in her dress that she wore to the funeral and without shoes, Penny stepped out of the vehicle and placed her bare feet on the rain-soaked pavement adjacent from the accident scene. She couldn't see the car involved because of the positioning of the emergency vehicles. Rescue workers scurried about, and Penny strained to see what was going on. Finally, soaked and desperate, she caught a glimpse of a headlight. It was encased in white and was approximately eight inches by ten inches. Penny recognized that headlight. She didn't need to see any more. Dean's aunt and uncle realized what had just occurred and immediately helped Penny back into their car to return her to Dean's memorial dinner.

Shortly after departing the scene of the accident, Penny received a phone call from the Highway Patrol asking her to come down to the hospital—the same hospital where Dean had recently passed away. Upon arriving, Penny was escorted to a small room and approached by a patrolman.

"Would you like to ID the body?"

Nobody can ever be prepared to be asked that question, especially after just leaving a funeral. While awaiting Penny's response, the patrolman handed her Michelle's driver's license. Staring down at the license, Penny simply responded, "No thank you. This is all I need." Penny's heart sank. She would have to go back to the dinner, the celebration of a beautiful life, and inform the guests that they had just lost another beautiful soul. Michelle was gone. Even in death, she and Dean couldn't be far apart from each other. Penny also had the arduous task of conveying this devastating news to all of her family, including Mom and Dad.

THE DAY OF DEAN'S FUNERAL, OCTOBER 6TH, 2005, WAS like any other fall day in North Dakota. The air had a significant chill to it, made worse by the occasional gusts of wind that was often present, giving subtle warning of the winter weather that would soon be returning for a near six-month stay. Standing out on our front porch and looking up at the cold, gray sky seemed to make the already chilly air appear significantly colder.

Moments later, I was joined by Mitzie on the porch. She was preparing to run to the local grocery store to pick up a few things for dinner.

"Wow, it's really starting to get cold out here," she said. She wrapped her arms around herself as if she was trying to give herself a hug and provide some additional warmth.

"Yeah, it almost feels as though there's a storm working its way in," I responded. We had lived in the northern plains long enough to have experienced sudden weather changes like this before, and we were pretty much able to predict impending snow storms with a fairly confident level of accuracy. October was always an unpredictable month in North Dakota. One day, it could be a warm fall day, and the next may give way to the wrath of an early winter.

After a long day at the police department, I was incredibly tired. Being the chief of a small-town department was stressful enough, but with Dean's funeral, this day had been a little extra trying. I was heavy in thought about my little sister, wondering how she was doing. Mitzie and I weren't able to make the near 2,000-mile trek down to Wilmington for his funeral because I was involved in a trial for a young man that had been arrested for various drug-related charges. Dean wasn't yet a relative of mine, so the judge wasn't willing to release me from my subpoena to attend the funeral. I couldn't blame him. This was an important case and needed to be tried without interruption. I was content knowing that Penny and her husband Ed were there with Michelle during this trying time in her life. I would wait for Michelle's phone call later on to learn all the details of the day and about Dean's funeral. Mainly, I just wanted to make sure she was doing okay.

Later that evening, my phone rang. I sat on my bed, reached for the phone, and held it to my ear, "Hello?"

"We've lost her." Penny's voiced echoed into the deep caverns of my thoughts. I vaguely recalled hearing those words and was incredibly confused by what they could mean. It was Dean's funeral. Who could get lost at a funeral?

The words crackled through the phone that chilly October evening. I'll never forget those words as long as I live.

"What do you mean, we lost her?" I asked.

Penny told me that Michelle had just died in an automobile accident on a rain-soaked highway near the coast of North Carolina. Thirty-two years old and her life was over.

I couldn't believe what I was just told and could barely comprehend the information as it was being conveyed to me. Penny continued to tell me the sorted details of the accident and how she had been given Michelle's driver's license by the Highway Patrol officer. I clearly heard what Penny was saying to me, but I knew that I would have to confirm this for myself, so I hung up the phone with her and called the hospital. A pleasant lady answered on the other end.

"I'm calling from North Dakota about my sister, Michelle Keeling," I said.

By this time, Mitzie had joined me in our bedroom.

"Honey, I can't give any information about anyone who may be here, but I can put one of your relatives on the phone." She said.

"I just hung up with her, that's why I'm calling you."

"Honey, I apologize but, I can't tell you anything."

I couldn't help but notice that the tone in her voice had changed, and her words softened in a more sympathetic manner. During my law enforcement career, I've interviewed many people for various things, ranging from criminal to tragedy, and I've heard this tone before.

"You just did." I replied.

I dropped the phone and immediately crouched to the floor, sobbing helplessly. Mitzie knelt down beside me and placed her arms around me, trying to provide as much comfort as she could. Everything became foggy, and I was having a difficult time compartmentalizing the news that had just enveloped my heart.

———

I WAS UNSURE WHETHER MITZIE AND I WOULD BE ABLE to get any real sleep that night. The shock that I was feeling was quickly replaced with a concern for Mom and Dad. What must it be like at their apartment at this very moment? I just couldn't imagine. It was all still so raw, and neither of my parents had the best coping skills in regards to receiving bad news. My siblings and I had lost our baby sister, but our parents had lost one of their children. I've never lost a child, thank God. I couldn't imagine what that must feel like. I would think that the only thing that could be worse would be either seeing it happen or hearing it happen. I could feel my body literally shaking as I thought about mom's phone call with Penny. Our poor mother heard her youngest child die. I felt my heart physically ache.

I knew that I had to get a hold of Mom and Dad soon. Mitzie was deep in the process of packing our bags and arranging our impending journey from North Dakota to Ohio. There were so many things to do. So many phone calls to make, but it was getting late into the evening, and I knew that I needed some rest. I forced myself to the quiet, dark confines of our bedroom in an attempt to get some sleep.

The following morning, I felt as though I had experienced a prize fight the night before. I was groggy and nearly every part of my body ached. I was still in disbelief over the accident that claimed my sister. As I slowly began to awaken from my slumber, all the emotions from the previous evening were also awoken. I knew that I couldn't allow these intense emotions to overtake me and completely occupy my thoughts. After all, I still hadn't had the chance to talk with my parents. I began transitioning from doldrums of sadness to the role of family caretaker, a role that I was used to.

After getting myself together and nearly stumbling as I got out of bed, I made my way down the creaky oak stairs to the kitchen for some coffee. Mitzie sat at the table talking with a school representative, trying to explain why Nicky and Jared wouldn't be attending for the next week or so. The kids sat quietly in the living room watching television. While pouring myself a cup of some much-needed coffee, I felt a slight nudge to my lower leg, causing me to nearly spill some blazing hot contents onto the floor. Directing my attention downward, I saw Skeeter Pete sitting patiently beside me. We had originally gotten her for the boys, but she quickly took to me and became my buddy. I enjoyed having her around. Faithful to a fault; she continued to stare up at me with her big brown eyes, waiting for me to return the bump she had just given me. It was almost as if she knew about the events that had recently transpired. Smiling, I leaned down and pet her on the head.

"What's up Skeeter Pete?" I asked.

We may have only had her for a little over a year, but she had clearly cemented herself as a member of our family. We loved her.

As I sipped on my coffee, I knew that my first phone call of the day would be with Mom. I didn't know exactly how our conversation would go or if she would even be willing to get on the phone with me, but now was the time to try. I picked up the phone and dialed her number.

"Mom, are you okay?" I softly asked.

I wasn't sure what sort of response I would get. I was pretty much preparing myself for just about anything. I didn't know if she would cry, scream, attempt to carry on a somewhat normal conversation, or simply hang up the phone.

"Oh, about as good as can be, I guess," she replied.

The pain and hurt were audible. I wanted so desperately to reach out and give her a hug. We were all hurting, but Mom's hurt seemed to be that much more. Her pain compounded mine.

"I don't know how we're gonna get her up here for a funeral," Mom continued.

It was a simple statement, but knowing her the way I did, it was actually a request. A quiet, somewhat desperate plea to do whatever I could in order to get Michelle's body transported from Wilmington to Caldwell. This was a question she didn't even need to ask. Mitzie and I were already planning on helping in any way we could with the arrangements.

"Don't even worry about it," I told her. "Let us take care of this."

Almost excitedly, she asked, "You sure you guys can help?" Her sobs were an unbearable release of emotion. Of course, I worry about both my parents, but there's something about Mom crying that nearly brought me to tears myself.

"I'll pay you back," she added.

I don't know why she even said that. Both of my parents were disabled and living on a fixed income. They could barely afford to keep their vehicle on the road, let alone attempt to take on a financial burden of this magnitude.

"Stop worrying, Mom. We'll bring Michelle home," I said.

After hanging up with her, Mitzie and Penny worked on the logistics of having Michelle prepared for a plane flight to Columbus. I knew that I now had the difficult task of calling my children, Amanda and Shawn, and letting them know about their Aunt Michelle. This would be tough. She was quite popular with her nieces and nephews, and they all loved her dearly.

While nearly all the children considered my brother Mike their favorite uncle, Michelle easily held the title of "favorite aunt." For Mike, it was because he was once a drummer in several rock bands, but for Michelle, it was because she happily spoiled each one of them, and allowed the kids to get away with just about everything. As a parent, I always cautioned her to not be so lenient, but as a person, I wished that I could have had an aunt just like her.

Denise and I always tried to be the cool ones, but could never seem to pull it off. We were more the disciplinarians and generally feared the children would get themselves hurt or come up missing if we failed to stay right on top of them. Mike and Michelle took a much different and more relaxed approach. I sometimes thought the kids were watching over *them* at times.

My heart broke as I listened to my daughter, Amanda, cry when I told her that Michelle had gone to be with the angels. I was hoping that her Aunt Patty was holding her and providing her with some comfort. There's absolutely no easy way to explain something like this to a fifteen-year-old child that worshipped the ground Michelle once walked on, but as her father, it was my job to do so. Once I finished talking with Amanda, I had to repeat this painful process with Shawn.

———

AFTER DROPPING SKEETER OFF AT A BOARDING KENNEL in Fargo, we began our long trek across the country. I've made this drive several times and was never a big fan of it. It was always a long trip, but this one felt so much longer. I had twenty-three hours or so to think about this tragedy and worry about Mom and Dad. We drove through the night, counting down each mile as if, somehow, that would make the trip shorter.

Early the following afternoon, Mitzie and I pulled into Crestwood Village, the apartment complex where Mom and Dad resided. The parking lot was nearly empty, but there were several people already scurrying. We had driven straight through the evening, only stopping for an occasional meal, restroom breaks, and to fill up with gas, and we were all completely exhausted. But I was with Mom and Dad now, and I was going to look after my parents. As much as I needed the sleep, it would simply have to wait.

Over the next couple of days, family members arrived and stopped in to see Mom and Dad. Everybody wanted to personally deliver their condolences, but I think Mom just wanted to be left alone. I couldn't blame her. Her entire existence had just recently been shattered. Mike and his wife, Carrie, arrived from Pennsylvania, and Penny and Ed drove up from North Carolina. Mitzie and I soon set out on another quick journey to pick up Amanda and Shawn. Strangely, all of this activity had the ambiance of a family reunion. Many friends and relatives milled around and hung out with each other, laughing, hugging, and generally spending moments talking about memories of Michelle. It seemed as though everyone had a special story to share. Michelle's funeral was planned for the upcoming Wednesday, so there was plenty of time to take care of all the details that typically accompany this type of event.

Mom really wanted a nice flower spray for Michelle's casket, but they were very expensive. Fresh flowers wouldn't last long, but she was persistent, and we knew we would have to find some way to make this happen. The night before the funeral, Mitzie, Penny, and Carrie drove to Walmart and purchased all the supplies necessary to make the highly requested flower arrangement. They worked tirelessly throughout the evening and made a stunningly beautiful display. Their work was made of artificial flowers and quickly assembled together, but this spray would rival any that could have been purchased.

The morning of Michelle's funeral started off like most regularly do. I dragged myself out of bed and made my way to mom's kitchen to enjoy a cup of coffee. As usual, Mitzie was already up, sitting at the dining room table, having a conversation with Penny. I was especially tired this morning. More tired than I normally was. We were up late the night before, continuing to catch up with relatives that were making their way into Caldwell to pay their respects.

I wasn't looking forward to this day at all. I knew that no matter how difficult it was going to be for us kids, it would surely be a little extra hard for Mom and Dad. Without a doubt, we would all need to be there for them and each other.

Slowly, everybody woke up, and the bathroom was a freight train of humanity making their way in and out as we showered, dressed, and prepared for the fairly full day that lay ahead of us. I had given this day considerable thought and dreaded its arrival. Up till now, we hadn't seen Michelle. Soon, we would all have the unwanted opportunity to do just that.

Mitzie and I, along with our children, left first for McVay-Perkins Funeral Home, followed shortly thereafter by Mike and Carrie. Penny and Ed were going to transport Mom and Dad, so they would leave last. I was amazed at how many vehicles were already at the funeral home when we got there. We climbed out of our Caravan and slowly made our way in to the building, our progress occasionally halted by well-wishers.

We quickly passed through the foyer and turned our attention toward the main area of the building. I paused momentarily before entering in to the viewing area. Mitzie signed the guest book for all of us and led the kids to the seating area. To my right, there was a large display board with seemingly a thousand pictures. It was a very nice photo display of Michelle through nearly every phase of her short life.

I noticed our cousin, Dwight, standing in front of the photo display intently observing each one, as if he were a detective scanning a photo lineup. I slowly made my way over to him to say hello, but as I got closer, I could see a long trail of tears making their way down his cheek. I wanted to offer him words of comfort that many had shared with me the past few days, but I also wanted him to have his moment.

After deciding to wait for a better time to have a conversation with Dwight, I finally turned around and directed my attention to Michelle. I could see her head propped up on a small white silk pillow. She looked so peaceful lying there under bright lights, on display for all in attendance to easily see. The beautiful flower arrangement that the girls had worked so feverishly on adorned her casket. True to her extreme NASCAR fandom, she was decked out in a bright orange shirt, displaying the number twenty, and the name of her favorite race car driver, Tony Stewart. I took notice of the heavy layers of makeup across her cheeks and up the bridge of her nose. This looked odd to me, because Michelle rarely wore makeup, except for very special occasions. This hardly felt like the special occasion you get dolled up for. Her death had suddenly become very real to me.

"Hey Chelle," I quietly said. My eyes welled up as I gently ran my hand over her shoulder.

Maybe it was because of the way she was laying. Perhaps it was because of the heavy impact of the crash, or maybe it was because it had been a few months since I had last seen her, but I couldn't help thinking that the person lying before me vaguely resembled my little sister. I felt Mitzie rubbing my lower back. I slowly turned to her, and she reached up and gave me a hug.

As we turned to walk away, I noticed that Penny and Ed had arrived with Mom and Dad. Shortly thereafter, Denise made her entrance. I knew deep down inside that the next few minutes were going to be painful. I mentioned to Mitzie that I was going to escort Mom up to the casket. As distraught as she was, I was unsure how she would handle seeing one of her children lying motionless in a casket. I quickly moved across the room and made my way toward the entrance to intercept my parents. I motioned for Mike and Penny to help me walk them up to Michelle.

Dad indicated that he would be fine and encouraged us to direct our attention toward our mother. I cradled one of her arms in an escort position while Penny held the other, and we began our slow walk toward the casket. It was only a short distance across the room, but it felt like an extremely long walk. As we approached Michelle, I could feel the weight of our mother increasing. Her legs got a bit wobbly, and her crying was becoming noticeably distinct. When we finally reached the casket, we slowly let go of mom's arms and she immediately reached out and touched Michelle's face.

With tears flowing like small streams helplessly to the floor, Mom leaned over and embraced Michelle, laying her head across Michelle's chest. After a couple of minutes, we told Mom that it was time to take a seat because the service would soon begin. As we began to turn Mom away from Michelle, she grasped the side of the casket with a grip much like a parent attempting to prevent a small child from running into traffic. We were forced to peel her fingers away from the casket to prevent it from tipping. After some effort, we were able to walk Mom a few feet back to her seat.

As I took my seat next to Mitzie, I recalled the various funerals that I had attended throughout my life. I remembered times sitting in the back of a room, much like this one, watching relatives of mine sitting in front of a loved one for a service. As I grew older, my seat, that was once in the back of the room, slowly advanced closer to the front row. Now, here I was, directly in front of a lost loved one while younger relatives sat quietly in the back of the room.

It was a beautiful service, invoking emotions from everyone in attendance. I really sympathized with Penny and Ed. It was a little less than a week prior that they were going through this very same process in North Carolina with Dean's funeral. Mike provided the soundtrack for the funeral, complete with many of Michelle's favorite songs, including "Daddy's Hands." She often sang that song to our father. Our cousin Charlie, Dwight's older brother, opened up the service with a short, heartfelt message before handing it off to Reverend Hoover, who officiated the formal proceedings.

Once finished, we all lined the streets of Caldwell, Ohio with our vehicles and began our long, slow procession to the cemetery. It was a cloudy day, in the low seventies, with a slight, but distinctly noticeable breeze in the air. I wondered to myself if it was going to rain with the way the clouds darkened above us. They threatened to add another layer of gloom to the day.

Sitting alongside my siblings and parents, under a dark green canopy, I found myself watching my twin sister, Denise. She was really hurting and seemed to be in a steady flow of tears since Michelle's accident. My heart ached for her.

Everyone made a final pass before Michelle was to be laid to rest, and I thought about all the times that Michelle had moved from town to town and state to state, and now she would finally come to rest in a country cemetery, on a wooded hill, outside Dudley, Ohio. Life was over for Michelle, but those hands on the clock keep ticking.

6

LIFE AFTER MICHELLE

The following day, a small group of us ventured to a restaurant in Cambridge for a bite to eat. As we sat sharing memories and engaging in casual conversation, we were soon approached by a young waitress. Turning our attention toward her, we were suddenly amazed the person standing before us. She looked nearly identical to Michelle. As we all continued to rather rudely stare at this young waitress, and back and forth at each other, a look of confusion came over her.

"Is there anything wrong?" she asked.

"Oh my God," Penny blurted out. "I'm sorry for staring at you, but you closely resemble our little sister who recently passed away."

"You definitely do," I added. "Her name was Michelle."

Smiling back at us, the waitress said, "That's my name."

I could tell she was taken back a bit and was becoming somewhat nervous at the group of strangers suddenly comparing her to a lost relative. I'm almost positive that this wasn't something that she was expecting when she approached our table. Gathering herself, she quickly replied, "I'm so sorry for your loss. Can I get you started with some drinks?"

We finally came to our senses and ordered our drinks and meals. We spent the better part of the next hour enjoying some really good homemade food and each other's company. I knew that this would most likely be the last time we would all be together for the foreseeable future. While we finished up our dinners, I kept reflecting back to our waitress and her striking resemblance to our sister. I sat back and smiled while the others continued talking with one another. I don't believe in ghosts, spirits, or coincidences, but I do believe Michelle stopped in for a brief moment to let us know that she was going to be okay. It was a fleeting and confirming comfort before we went back to everyday life.

———

WE LEFT MOM AND DAD TO RETURN AMANDA AND Shawn back to Rose, and we started the drive back to North Dakota. Penny and Ed were well on their way back to Spring Lake, and Mike and Carrie were already safely back in Pennsylvania. Although they seemed to be doing well when we left, I was still quite concerned about my parents. My concern also extended toward Denise. I wished that I didn't have to leave so soon, although I firmly believed that Mom and Dad were ready for everyone to leave. I think they just wanted to get back to some sort of normal, whatever that would now be.

It would take Mitzie, Nicky, Jared, and I two full days to return to Mayville. Unlike the trip out to Ohio, we weren't in any hurry to get back. Periodically during our drive, I checked in with Mom and Dad. I wasn't leaving anything to chance. Mainly, I just needed to convince myself that they were going to be alright.

Once back in Mayville, I wanted to slide back into my normal routine. I was happy to return to the police department. I wanted to get back to the task of providing leadership to my officers and being a community leader to the residents. Mitzie returned to her job, although she was never really content. The boys got back to school and picked up exactly where they left off. Mostly, I just wanted to keep my mind occupied and not use so much energy thinking about Michelle.

I continued to reach out to Mom and Dad to see how things were going for them. For years, I had always felt it was my duty, as the oldest son, to be my family's protector, and this fell within my long list of duties. It appeared as though they were both doing fine and were actively moving on with their lives, at least initially. My father appeared to return to his normal daily activities somewhat quicker than Mom. He always loved to go fishing and would often spend countless hours on the shores of area lakes and rivers, mostly drowning worms and feeding the fish bits of corn and chicken livers. Occasionally, he would reel in a nice-sized catfish or a perch or two, but he had no interest in keeping them. Dad never really had an appetite for cleaning, preparing, or eating wild fish. He simply enjoyed fishing for the sport of it.

Mom always tried to give everyone the impression that she was successfully moving forward and not dwelling on Michelle's passing, but it became apparent that it was mostly a front. Nearly everyone that knew her could tell. She was struggling, quietly. She was crawling into her own private space and slowly segregating herself from her husband and the rest of her family. It would take me a while to realize the significance of her inactivity, but when I did, I had no idea of how to deal with it. More importantly, I had no idea how provide Mom with the help she clearly needed. Occasionally, she would reveal the cracks in her solidarity and share her struggles in bits and pieces during our phone calls. Without any prompting, she would sometimes utter, "I sure do miss Michelle."

Mom was mentally torturing herself, and sadly, I was allowing it to happen because I refused to discuss Michelle's accident. I didn't want to relive those tragic events and go through the emotional torment that I had felt during her memorial and funeral. For me, it was easier to just walk away from this topic every time it came up.

Mom wouldn't be alone in her personal struggles. Mike and Denise both had their moments where Michelle's death played a significant role in decisions that they would make in each of their lives. Penny would talk about the accident when asked to, but she mostly kept it to herself. We were all hurting and would continue to do so for years to come. For me, I wanted no part in discussing her accident, death, or memories for many years. My personal safe space was immersing myself into my work and refusing to look back.

———

SHORTLY AFTER RETURNING TO NORTH DAKOTA, MITZIE and I decided to return to Minot. This was due to better employment opportunities for her. Mayville was a pleasant town, and the residents welcomed us into their community, but we never seemed to feel at home there. We looked forward to getting back to Minot. Mitzie had previously worked for ING prior leaving for Mayville. She was able to maintain some really close friendships and a solid rapport with the management there. Going back to work at ING wasn't a difficult decision.

Mitzie and the boys left for Minot before me. They purchased a home, and with the assistance of her parents, re-established residency there. I remained behind to assist the city leaders in finding a new chief of police and go through the process of handing over the department. I joined my family in Minot a couple of months later.

I continued to work in the law enforcement field a few more years until the fall of 2010, when I made a complete career change and took a job with an oilfield service company as a crew dispatcher and trainer. Although I occasionally missed working as a police officer and serving the general public, I enjoyed the many challenges that the oil and gas industry offered. I also really appreciated the significantly higher wages that accompanied it.

Over the next couple years, we traveled back and forth to visit with my parents, and I could easily see that Mom wasn't adjusting well to life without Michelle. She was spending more and more time in her bed, essentially sleeping her days away. When she was no longer able to naturally sleep for long hours, she medicated herself to sleep. We were all becoming quite concerned because her doctors were also prescribing her many additional medications with stronger, more potent doses. I feared that I was witnessing my mother slowly killing herself. She was becoming someone that I barely recognized, and it was destroying me.

IT WASN'T UNTIL 2012 THAT I FINALLY OPENED UP AND discussed my sister's death. Of course, I didn't come to this newfound revelation entirely on my own. With a bit of coaxing from a friend of mine, I created a presentation and began sharing it with people all over. I used Michelle's accident as the basis for the presentation, specifically sharing the fact that she was distracted at the time of her accident. Perhaps I was hiding my pain from the loss of a loved one behind a carefully crafted message of being safe while driving a vehicle. However, I felt it was a win-win situation with everyone involved. It helped me significantly, by allowing me to open up and permit my penned-up sadness to escape. Those who attended the lecture received a personal message of the dangers of distracted driving. I had been holding it in for several years and speaking publicly about Michelle felt like I was taking a heavy weight off my shoulders. I felt like I could breathe again.

During my various travels, I had the opportunity to deliver what I aptly dubbed *Michelle's Story* to audiences. Occasionally, my journey brought me near my parents' home. I wanted so badly for both of them to attend one of those presentations, but Mom refused. She wanted no part in hearing about Michelle's accident, and she made it very clear each time I extended them an invitation. Dad never actually said no, but he also never made himself available to attend. After a couple attempts, their lack of desire to hear my presentation became evident, and I never invited them again. I would forever honor their wishes. Besides, who was I to try to force Mom and Dad to relive that horrific moment? I had spent years refusing to even mention it, let alone relive it.

As time moved forward, Mom and Dad continued to live their lives in relative isolation. It became increasingly obvious to us kids that they weren't taking very good care of themselves. They also began missing scheduled doctor's appointments. We were all worried about their wellbeing and began seeking various avenues of care for them. Mitzie and I decided that it would be best if we brought them out to our home, and we began making some plans for this.

In the fall of 2012, Mitzie and I were finally ready to move Mom and Dad out to North Dakota to live with us. We had recently built a new home, complete with five bedrooms and three bathrooms. We had plenty of room and only had to figure out the logistics of transporting two older people, who weren't exactly in the best of health, over eighteen hundred miles, with everything they owned in life. Soon, an opportunity presented itself, oddly enough, by way of another major storm making its way up the eastern seaboard. Hurricane Sandy wreaked havoc on northern New Jersey and New York City, causing massive flooding and damage to nearly everything in her path. The company that I worked for participated in a humanitarian mission to help remove the massive amounts of water out of the Manhattan and Newark areas. I was able to be a part of this rewarding venture. I spent approximately a week and a half working between New Jersey and New York City, and then I made my way to Mom and Dad's place to help them pack everything up and drive them out to Minot.

———

ONE THING I'VE LEARNED OVER THE YEARS IS, THE drive from Ohio to North Dakota is extremely long in a car, but when you're in a long, fully loaded U-Haul truck, with three adults sitting side by side, the trip feels twice as long. To add to the discomfort, Mom was incredibly sick on the day we departed. She seemed to get much worse as the trip went along. A couple of times during the drive, I feared that we would have to stop and take her to a hospital. Being as stubborn as she was, Mom made me continue to drive and made every attempt to assure my father and I that she was going to be okay and not to worry about her. She just wanted to get the trip over with.

Shortly after arriving home, Mom was hospitalized with a rather severe blood infection. When she was transported to the emergency room, the doctors essentially placed her in a medically induced coma. She was very sick. Had Mitzie and I not decided to move them in with us, Mom would have probably died. The reality of her situation broke my heart. As difficult as the trip was on her physically, it was the right move.

Mom spent the better part of the next two weeks in the hospital. The majority of that time was in ICU. We saw her daily, having to wear gowns, gloves, and masks to prevent the spread of the infection. After she was released, she visited a doctor daily, for forty-one straight days, to receive an intravenous antibiotic infusion. This process took nearly an hour each time she went. We felt so lucky that we had caught the infection and that we could get her the treatment that she needed; however, we were all surprised that she had gotten so sick.

Time moved forward, and we tried to make my parents as

comfortable as possible and help them feel more at home. Dad was growing increasingly restless and was missing his life back home. He had never before ventured far from West Virginia. In fact, he had spent his entire life between West Virginia, Ohio, and Pennsylvania, and now I had him living a half a country away in North Dakota. Mom seemed to be a bit more at ease, but had come to rely on sleeping pills in an effort to sleep her days away. Her addiction to these sleep aids were becoming more and more worrisome until Mitzie and I finally decided to take control of her medications and administer them as they were prescribed. We also carefully checked her bedroom periodically to make sure she wasn't hiding any pills for later consumption. Nearly every time we checked, we found something hidden under her mattress or in a dresser drawer. It broke my heart that we had to do this. I felt like a prison guard conducting random cell shakedowns. These searches and the controlling of medications didn't sit well with Mom. There were many times when it sounded as though Mom hated Mitzie and I for restricting her medications. As hurtful as this was, we both realized that it was the addiction doing the talking and not her. Every day, I wished that I could reach deep into her soul and pull those demons out that were controlling her entire world. I wanted so badly to rid her of the pain.

During this time, my parents rarely got along with each other. At times I would blame myself, because it was my idea to move them so far away from their familiar surroundings. They were literally plucked out of their normal existence and inserted into a life that was very foreign to them. Mitzie and I were dealing with a great deal of stress at this point. Not only were we both working full-time jobs and taking care of Nicky, but we had also brought my daughter Amanda, and her son Brayden to Minot. A large portion of my job required me to travel out of state to different locations nationwide. I felt terrible flying away and leaving all this confusion for Mitzie to deal with on her own. I soon elected to change my job title within my company to one that would keep me home and not require me to travel nearly as much. God bless Mitzie! Not only did we nearly empty our savings to make all of this happen, but through it all, she somehow remained positive and kept a smile on her face. I knew she was crying on the inside.

The dynamics in our home were changing considerably as well. A home that once had plenty of space was now suddenly quite crowded, and at times, tempers would flare, and everyone's patience would run low. It was obvious that we weren't going to be able to maintain this existence for long.

A couple of months later, Amanda and her estranged husband seemed to have mended their fences and were talking on the phone several times a day. She soon began inquiring about how or when she and Brayden would be able to return to her home. It was about the same time when Dad began to hint around that he wanted to go back east, and he began formulating a plan to stay with his sister, Mary Ann, near Mannington, West Virginia. As much as I disliked the idea, and as expensive as I knew it was going to be, I eventually agreed to drive Dad, Amanda, and Brayden back to West Virginia. Logistically, it all worked out. Amanda was living in Philippi, and Aunt Mary Ann was living near Mannington. They were only separated by approximately fifty miles.

After getting Dad and Amanda loaded, I once again set out to venture across the country. By this time, Dad's health was declining a bit due to the onset of COPD. He could only walk a short distance before having to stop and catch his breath. I felt bad for him. I couldn't imagine how frightening it must be to lose your ability to breathe easily. We all encouraged him to stop smoking, but he continued to indulge in his lifelong habit.

It would be late in the evening when we finally pulled into Philippi. The weather was much different than what we had left behind in North Dakota. Although very cool and refreshing, compared to the northern plains, it felt like summer to me. As tired as I was after driving nearly twenty-four hours, I was thrilled with the prospect to see my son Shawn. With all the confusion that I had been experiencing lately, this was definitely a bonus for me. I missed that boy terribly and didn't get to see him often enough since he had entered adulthood. I assisted Amanda with unloading her and Brayden's belongings, gave them both a hug and a kiss, and Dad and I continued our journey to Mannington.

We arrived at Aunt Mary Ann's a short time later. I hadn't seen her in several years, and it was nice to have this opportunity to visit with her. More importantly, it would be nice to simply rest a couple days before beginning that arduous trek back across the country. While there, I took some time to refill my senses.

I trekked up the very same hill that my father had grown up on, in that tiny cabin that he had often spoken so fondly of. Sitting up on the hill, away from everyone, I was able to rest my mind from all the stress that I had been subjecting myself to. North Dakota and time had drowned some of my memories, and I had forgotten just how therapeutic it was to simply breathe in some mountain air and listen to the various noises that emanated from the dark reaches of the woods. The noises were both relaxing and haunting, but they were some much-needed medicine for my soul. I took in the intoxicating air and hoped it would fuel me for some time.

By the time I got back to Minot, the weather had begun to get a bit better. Spring began to settle into the northern plains. The sun was shining and temperatures began to rise, but you can never really put total faith in the weather remaining that way for long. Spring represents new beginnings. With only Mom left at the house, Mitzie and I hoped we could help her as she continued her difficult journey toward healing. But early spring can be unpredictable, with surprise snowstorms striking at any moment.

For some time, Mom showed signs that she was returning to her normal self. I relished in those moments, because I was growing weary and increasingly restless over her tremendous sorrow. There were times when she would smile, laugh, and outwardly enjoy normal everyday activities, such as going out to dinner with us. Then, there were other times when she would withdraw and crawl back into the depths of her despair. This became evident when we would go into her room while she slept. I would often see her lying on her side, facing a photograph of Michelle and Dean that sat on her nightstand at eye level. I envisioned her lying there, staring at this picture, and crying herself to sleep. As bad as I felt seeing her lie there, I was somewhat comforted that she was sleeping and not hurting; for a few hours, at least.

Dad seemed to be doing well. Mike had moved him from Aunt Mary Ann's home to Pennsylvania to be near him and Carrie. Shortly after arriving, Mike helped Dad get an apartment, and he was soon living on his own and caring for himself. Everyone was so proud and happy for him, especially Mom. She and Dad would often talk on the phone with each other, and it was easy to see that another long-distance move was on the horizon.

As spring turned to summer, Mom discussed returning to Pennsylvania and continuing her life together with Dad. I couldn't have been more thrilled with the progress Dad was making by living on his own, or with the fact that he and Mom were getting along much better than they had in quite some time, however I was very apprehensive about her moving so far away from Mitzie and I. We had finally been able to get her health back in a positive direction and were able to regulate her medications. I also couldn't help thinking about her near-death experience when she first came to live with us.

Regardless of what we thought about the idea of her departing, Mom wanted to go live with her husband, and she set her sights back east. I'm not entirely sure if it was one of her best qualities or if she was just a stubborn person, but when Mom would get her mind set on something, she would usually follow through with it.

It was June 2013, when Mike flew out to Minot to drive a U-Haul truck, packed full of Mom and her belongings, back to Pennsylvania. As Mitzie and I said our tearful goodbyes, I could sense some hesitation from Mom, but after all the planning and considerable costs associated with this move, she would head back east to resume her life with Dad.

———

MOM AND DAD SETTLED INTO A QUAINT APARTMENT that was perfect for low income or fixed income families. Initially, they seemed to be doing rather well, but it wouldn't be long before they would get back into their old routines. Mom had begun spending large portions of her days in bed sleeping, and Dad continued to allow it. On several occasions, Mike would take time from work to shuttle them to and from medical appointments and for groceries, but they would cancel their appointments or find some random reason not to go. I guess some demons are just too powerful to fight, and depression was that unyielding demon for Mom.

A few months later, my parents decided to, once again, move and share a residence with Mom's sister, Carol, and her family. Their reasoning for sharing household expenses made some sense, but I felt strongly that this decision was a bad idea.

———

THE RINGING CELL PHONE SHOOK ME FROM MY regular routine. I recognized the number and thought Mom was calling to talk, which was something she was doing quite often. I always loved talking with her, but our recent phone calls were mainly her wishing she had never left our home. My heart would break as I sat with the phone up to my ear, listening to her cry as she described her current situation.

"Hello?" I asked, not really knowing if I was going to get happy Mom or sad Mom. It came as a bit of a surprise to hear Dad's voice on the other end. Dad and I were barely talking at this time. Wrong or right, I placed blame on him for the current predicament they found themselves in. The only time Dad picked up the phone to call me was when something was wrong with Mom.

"Hey, Dennis?" He stuttered, almost as if he was going to ask me a question.

"Yeah, what's up?" I returned.

"Your mom is on her way to the hospital," he continued. "She fell and hit her face on the floor."

Convinced that she was going to be okay, and that this was just another trip, that she had made before for minor medical care, I asked Dad to keep me informed and I immediately called Mike.

"Yeah, I'm heading that way now," he said.

I wasn't overly concerned, and I was content to simply sit back and await my brother's phone call, informing me that Mom was going to be okay.

———

I COULD CLEARLY HEAR THE WORDS COMING OUT OF MY brother's mouth and being channeled through the speaker in my cell phone, but they didn't seem to be registering in my brain. Perhaps I was just refusing to believe what I was being told. I had convinced myself that she was going to be fine, but that's not the message Mike was relaying.

"It's not looking good," Mike said with a somber tone in his voice. "They ran a bunch of tests and found something. I'll have the doctor call you," he continued.

How can this be? She simply fell and hit her face. My thought process led me to believe that she would have a bump on her head, or at worst, a broken nose. Surely it couldn't be any worse than that. What did he mean by, "It doesn't look good?"

I continued visualizing Mom, lying in a hospital bed. I'd seen her in one before. I had talked about her health with the attending physician before. I was running a bunch of random questions through my mind, trying to make sense of this sudden event, but deep down inside my heart, I knew how this was going to end. Much like Michelle's accident, I just needed some confirmation. Soon, that confirmation would come with the ringing of another phone call. Looking intently at my screen, I stared at the unrecognized Pennsylvania number. My heart sank when I pressed the green circle on my screen.

"Hello?" I asked. Before anyone answered on the other end, I'm sure the tone of my voice gave a clear impression of the sadness and utter despair I was currently experiencing.

"Hi, is this Dennis?" the voice on the other end asked. His voice was deep. It had the sound of a person who spoke with both command and empathy. I was very confident that this doctor was about to give me news that I wasn't ready to hear. Gathering myself, I quickly responded, "Yes, it is."

The doctor explained to me that, due to her fall, they had pretty much conducted a full body scan to search for additional injuries. During this process, they located a large lump near her abdomen and immediately took her into surgery to remove it. Tears rolled down my face as the authoritative voice in my phone continued to explain to me that they were unable to remove the lump, and she wouldn't survive. My mother was dying, and I had to somehow come to terms with this.

"Your mother has a standing order to not be kept on any sort of lifesaving equipment," he said.

I knew Mom never wanted to be hooked up to anything in order to extend her life. She had always made this abundantly clear with all of us kids, and now, I knew that I was going to have to violate her final wishes in order to allow enough time for Mitzie and I to fly out and see her before she died. With a simple request, the doctor agreed to leave her breathing tube in.

———

IT HAD BEEN MANY YEARS SINCE I LAST DROVE INTO Coudersport. Mitzie and I were tightly packed into an extremely small rental car that we had picked up at the airport in Pittsburgh. She had called ahead and reserved us a room at a hotel immediately across the street from the hospital. This was the same hospital that mom had given birth to us kids a lifetime ago. There wasn't much in this small mountain town, but we weren't there for sightseeing.

We pulled into the parking lot at the hospital and walked into the main entrance. We made our way to Mom's floor and stepped out of the elevator. I started getting that familiar ache in my stomach from the anticipation of not knowing what I was going to see. Penny, who had arrived sometime earlier, approached us and led us back to Mom's room. Looking down at her, I was instantly taken back to the time, a couple years previously, when I watched her lay in a hospital bed, similar to the one she was in now. The wires and tubes, the beeps and drips were all familiarly hooked up to her. I wanted so badly to cry, but I couldn't. I needed to be a strong front and help my family through this. I slowly approached the side of her bed.

"Hey, Mom. How ya doing?" I asked.

Her eyes were closed, and I wasn't sure she could even hear me. I reached out and ran my hand over her silver hair. Slowly, her eyes opened. She stared up at me as if she was trying to figure out who I was.

"Mitzie is here too," I said, as Mitzie stepped closer.

"Hey Gail," she said.

Mom's blank stare was suddenly replaced by a confused look. I could tell she was trying to determine why both of us were in Pennsylvania, standing at her bedside. Turning her head, she scanned the room, which was now occupied by Penny, Denise, Aunt Rosie, Mitzie, me. Mike was on his way from his home in Johnsonburg. As quickly as her eyes had opened, they closed nearly as fast, and she drifted back off to sleep. Bending down, I gave her a kiss on her forehead and slowly exited the room.

The next few days were rather busy and mostly a blur for me. A small group of us had commandeered an adjoining room, just off the waiting area, and turned it in to our own personal headquarters. Many of our relatives and people that I hadn't seen in quite some time made their way to see Mom and visit with everyone hanging around in the waiting area. Ronda and Juny were making daily visits and bringing food for those of us who were maintaining a vigil over mom. We were becoming increasingly exhausted with the long hours and intermittent sleep. Mitzie and I shared our room with Penny and Denise so everyone could get rest in shifts.

As the week continued moving forward, we could see the changes in Mom's appearance as she neared her impending death. Watching someone you love go through the end of life is intensely heartbreaking. There is nothing you can do to prevent it.

One glimmering light in all of this sorrow was one of Mom's nurses that tended to her. His name was Kevin, and this man was a saint. One evening, as he was going off shift, he stopped in to Mom's room to let us know that he was going to be off for the next couple days and wished us well. He then leaned over and kissed our mother on the forehead. It was one of the sweetest moments I have ever witnessed from a healthcare provider, and it also signaled to me that Mom was very close to dying, and he knew it. He didn't have to tell us. His actions spoke loud and clear.

A short time later, I left to get some rest. I don't think I was away longer than a half hour when my phone rang. It was Mitzie, and she was delivering the news that I knew was coming. I still wasn't ready for it.

"She's gone," she said. I could hear her trying to speak as she choked back tears. She knew that I was going to be devastated.

"I'll be right over," I replied. I might have said that I would be right over, but it was going to take me a bit longer than that. I sat on the edge of the bed, supporting my head in my palms, allowing the tears to track down my face. For many years, I had always thought of myself as my family's protector, but at this moment, I was a son who had just lost his mother. I wasn't able to protect anyone from this.

I slowly walked back to the hospital to join Mitzie and Penny. I looked down at Mom's face, and I couldn't help but think of just how peaceful she appeared. Fighting back some more tears, I smiled slightly. I hadn't seen her look this way in many years. There would be no more need to cry herself to sleep, or to relentlessly push the pain away with her sorted medications. Instead, it was time for her to rest easy. Her single greatest wish had finally come true. She was once again going to see Michelle. Slowly, I bent down and kissed her on the forehead as Kevin had earlier. Quietly, I whispered in her ear, "Tell her I said hello when you get there."

I had so many mixed feelings surging through me. I was obviously grieving the loss of my mother, but part of me rejoiced that Mom wasn't going to hurt any longer. Part of me was sad that my brother, sisters, and I had lost out on ten years with our mother. She just couldn't get past Michelle's death, and because of her debilitating depression, she shut herself down and gave up on ever being happy again. But she finally was released from the wicked grasp of such a horrible mental illness. We may have lost a mother, but heaven gained another angel. I was okay with that.

7

THE BEGINNING DAYS OF SHARING MICHELLE'S STORY

I wasn't ever planning on sharing my sister's story with others. I rarely talked about her accident. In fact, I rarely discussed her death with anyone, including family members. I couldn't fathom the idea of disclosing something so personal with perfect strangers. I was quite content simply keeping it to myself. I kept her tragedy safely tucked away in my personal archives of memories, and I only brought it out when it was convenient and I was ready. True, I was being greedy with her memory, but I figured it was nobody's business that my little sister had perished on a highway in eastern North Carolina nearly seven years earlier. Sadly, I wasn't seeing the bigger picture, and I wasn't hearing the true message. With the help of a dear friend, the deeper meaning of sharing such a personal event with others would soon become much clearer. The memories surrounding the creation of Michelle's story were both somewhat frightening and pleasant at the same time. Some events in a person's life are as vivid and memorable as they were the day they occurred. Making the decision to put *Michelle's Story* together will always be one of those moments for me. I often look back fondly at the time I began a relatively small and somewhat routine project that would eventually lead me on a personally challenging and heartfelt journey around the country.

It was late spring in 2012 when the earliest thoughts of sharing Michelle's story first presented itself. Nearly four years before Mom's passing. I appreciated the freedom of being able to work independently and enjoyed training and mentoring fellow employees. I really loved my job, even though the oil and gas industry can be extremely volatile and changes often.

One day, while sitting in my office, I received a phone call from the VP of environmental health and safety, Kelly George. It wasn't all that unusual for Kelly to call me. A year previously, he had personally recruited me for an open safety position, and from that point on, we seemed to get along well. Over time, we became friends that would often bounce ideas off each other. His friendship and leadership meant a lot to me, so when he called to discuss things with me, I listened intently. This call, however, came with a request, a request that I didn't see coming.

After exchanging pleasantries, as we always did, Kelly began discussing our upcoming safety conference that was going to take place later in the summer in Bakersfield, California. At some point in time during the conversation, the subject of distracted driving came up, mainly because of all the vehicle incidents that our company had been experiencing. My previous career in law enforcement was also considered, but this subject garnered images and thoughts of a painful chapter in my life. After all, distracted driving was one of the contributing factors to Michelle's automobile accident.

"Do you think you could come up with something to present at the conference?" Kelly asked.

"I'm sure I can," I hesitantly replied.

"Okay then, prepare some things and send them to me. I'll give ya a call later," he said.

Once our phone call ended, I knew that if I were going to do a presentation, it was going to be about the dangers of distracted driving. With this in mind, I knew that I was going to have to prepare myself to talk about Michelle's death, something that I had carefully kept embedded deep inside me. As I sat back in my office chair, chewing on the end of my pen, I closed my eyes and tentatively opened up my mental library and slowly pulled Michelle's volume off the shelf.

After some thought and reflection, I opened up my laptop and began typing. With a couple of hastily constructed paragraphs, consisting of several spelling and grammatical errors, I briefly introduced Kelly to my sister. This would become the beginning of a very long and rewarding journey that Michelle and I would go on together. I had no way of knowing exactly how many miles we would travel together while sharing this story, or just how many people we would ultimately stand in front of while delivering it. All I knew was this accident contained a story and a message that needed to be shared, and Kelly had provided me with the means to do just that.

The greatest lesson my mentor had taught me was to never let an incident go to waste, no matter how devastating it may have been. It was time for me to stop running from my personal grief. It was time for me to use Michelle's story to hopefully help others that may find themselves in similar situations or may have lost someone that they cared a lot about. Oddly enough, this request had provided me with an unusual level of motivation.

Most people say that one of the scariest things they've ever done is to speak in public. It wasn't singing in front of people. Not even heights. Somehow public speaking had found its way to the top of the list. For me, being an OSHA instructor, and a former law enforcement trainer, I had plenty of experience speaking in front of people, and I wasn't necessarily bothered by it. I was rather comfortable talking to any group, large or small.

From entry level to upper management. It didn't really matter to me. The scariest part for me was knowing it would force me to finally deal with her death, which, till then, was something I had always refused to do. There was always a convenient excuse for me to not talk about it, but as painful as it would be, I realized it needed to be done. I was going to rise up to this challenge.

Over the next couple of weeks, I carefully put together a presentation that consisted of a dozen or so slides. Some of these slides contained pictures of Michelle's destroyed car, her tombstone, and a picture of her and Dean. The presentation was approximately twenty minutes in length, but once finished, I wasn't entirely sure whether I could deliver it. There were a couple times when I nearly backed out of my obligation to speak at the conference. I didn't want to force myself to look back and be subjected to those painful feelings that I had strategically hidden for so many years, but I knew that deep down inside, this would be the beginning of a healing process that I had always neglected to offer myself. I teared up often just practicing it, but a commitment was a commitment, and I wasn't going to back out on this one. I worked diligently until I could recite the presentation with very little difficulty. Finally, I attached the presentation and some notes to an email and sent it off to California for approval.

———

Sitting on the plane, from Denver to Bakersfield, I continuously rehearsed my presentation silently in my head, and I envisioned myself standing in front of strangers belting out each line. I don't know if I was more nervous about presenting Michelle's story for the very first time or if I was simply being apprehensive about finally sharing it publicly. Regardless, Kelly already had a copy of the presentation, and I was on the agenda.

Later that evening, while sitting in my room at the Double Tree off Rosedale Highway, I continued to go over my presentation. At times, I would get up and pace back and forth as I rehearsed it. Why was I so nervous? After all, I've delivered literally hundreds of presentations in the past. But this wasn't just another presentation. This wasn't some canned safety training. No, this one was very personal to me, and I needed to do it justice. Part of me was looking forward to sharing her story, while another part of me wished that I would have never agreed to participate.

I knew that I would have a difficult time getting a full night's sleep, but I had to try. Lying on the bed, a couple of thoughts kept swirling in my mind.

I hope this goes well. This has to be the most uncomfortable bed I've ever laid on.

I didn't even remember falling asleep when the faint, familiar sound of my cell phone forced my eyes open and with it, a new day. Mitzie signaled me that it was time to get up and prepare myself for this very important day. I always loved hearing her voice in the morning as I woke up, especially when I was on the road. By this time, Mitzie and I had been together for fourteen years. During this time, I had traveled often, and her early morning phone calls never grew old. Rubbing the sleep from the corners of my eyes, I slowly reached across the nightstand and picked up my phone. Pressing the button and placing it to my ear, I quietly asked, "Hello?"

"Rise and shine, baby!" she said.

Mitzie was always a morning person, and as usual, she was very chipper when she would make her calls. It always makes me smile to hear her voice. She has a knack for getting my days off to a good start.

"I'm up," I replied.

Knowing me as well as she did by this point, she knew that this was a big day for me and that I would surely be nervous about it. You wouldn't be able to tell by the sound of her voice. Right now, I really needed her encouragement and positive thoughts.

"Good luck today. You're gonna do great!" she said, in her usual reassuring voice.

———

FOR THE OTHERS ATTENDING THIS CONFERENCE, IT may have just been another day, another gathering, but for me, it was so much more. I showered, dressed, and made my way down to the hotel restaurant to have some coffee and breakfast. I robotically ran the details of my presentation through my head as I slowly crunched through a piece of toast with a generous amount of grape jelly on it.

After finishing my breakfast and a quick scan of the morning paper, I walked back to my room to gather some items that I would be taking with me to our safety conference.

Kelly had arranged for a couple of vans to be at the hotel to shuttle me and my colleagues to the conference room a continental five miles away. I had been in Bakersfield a couple times and I was still amazed at how fast the traffic appeared to be flowing. I was certainly happy that I didn't have to drive through the mess. A few minutes later, we pulled up to the parking area where our company was headquartered. One by one, we exited the vehicles and walked through a gated area toward the building. It almost felt like we were children arriving at school for the first day.

Once in the building, I perused the room for people that I knew. Everyone in attendance either knew each other or knew of each other, so there really weren't any strangers, but we only saw each other once a year. I made sure that I sat next to the safety coordinator at our Pennsylvania branch, Rich. We had met approximately a year earlier here in Bakersfield, at an event much like this one and had become pretty good friends. I always enjoyed Rich's sense of humor. He had a heavy New York accent and reminded me of someone you might find hanging out on the streets of Brooklyn.

After securing a cup of boiling hot coffee, I made my way around the room, shaking hands and engaging in casual conversation with the other attendees. I was just trying to get as comfortable as I possibly could with everyone before my time came to tell them a very personal story. Soon, Kelly entered the room and everyone took their seats, so the day of presentations and information sharing could begin.

"Welcome," Kelly said.

Kelly had a noticeable habit of rubbing his hands together when he talked, and he always had a slight smirk on his face. You never really knew what he was thinking, and he was often full of surprises. He appeared to be very comfortable in front of a room of people and beamed with confidence as he spoke. Pacing the room slightly, he made small talk by asking how everyone's trip to California had gone, then he meticulously reviewed the event agenda that we would be following for the next couple days. He had a casual way of carrying himself and was well spoken and rather easy to listen to. As nervous as I was about my portion of this conference, I was equally excited to hear the other presentations and learn some things from each of them.

Throughout the day, Kelly went through the different topics listed on his agenda, one after another. Thankfully, most of them were participatory, which made staying alert much easier. He kept the event structured, but he also created an environment that allowed all of us to remain comfortable and engaged. Whenever we had a small break and when we stopped for lunch, I revisited and studied my presentation notes; as if I was somehow going to forget the details. Slowly, I was able to calm myself down and was becoming a little less nervous about speaking. Now, I just had to wait until it was my turn.

The speaker before me was a man named David. He worked at one of our locations in Colorado and had a relaxed demeanor as he spoke. Stoically, he described a series of events that led to a near explosion that had almost taken his life years earlier while at work. Watching him talk, you could visibly see his story's effects on his face. With tears in his eyes and his hands shaking, he relived every single detail of that terrible event. I felt so bad for him. He was truly a lucky man to have survived that day, and by sharing his story, he was not allowing the incident go to waste, as Kelly had often reminded each of us to never do. After he was finished talking, I was brought back to reality. It was my turn.

As I made my way to the front of the room, the anxiety that I had been experiencing while preparing *Michelle's Story* fully resurfaced. I could feel my throat drying, and I began to sweat slightly.

"Come on Dennis, get it together," I whispered to myself.

Shaking slightly and holding the laser pointer in my increasingly wet palms, I began to talk about distracted driving and share my sister's story. The more I talked, the more the events of that tragic day came flooding back to me. Periodically, I had to refocus and restrain the emotions that I had nearly allowed to escape on a couple of occasions. Much like David before me, I was sure it was apparent that this story was extremely difficult for me to share. The look on everyone's face told me that I had their attention. I continued through the presentation, and once finished, I let out a large breath, as if I had been holding it in the entire time. Walking back to my seat, several of the attendees shared their condolences for my loss and thanked me for telling the story of Michelle's untimely death. I found myself suddenly overtaken by another completely different set of emotions. I had made it through that moment that I had seemingly dreaded for so long. I did it. I had conquered that fear and had crossed a significant bridge in my healing process. Little did I know then that this would only be the beginning. There would be so much more that I would get to experience. It wouldn't be until later that evening that I would realize the full impact that Michelle's story had on my audience. As a group of us sat in the hotel lounge, enjoying a few cocktails, several of my colleagues shared with me their thoughts about my presentation and asked me to share more details about her accident. A few offered up similar stories about people they knew that had also lost their lives in vehicle accidents. Listening to each of them talk, I knew that sharing this story was the right thing to do, as difficult as it was. Her death was no longer going to be a greedily guarded tragedy. I felt that her story would help others heal. I wouldn't let her life and tragic death be wasted.

Never let an incident go to waste.

———

Back in Minot, I refined my presentation and considered sharing it with others. I remembered the conversations that I had had with the people back in Bakersfield and really felt that the story may have had some sort of impact and may have resonated with them. I kept thinking that sharing Michelle's story could save lives. If it could reach one person and help him or her think before picking up their phone while driving, then I should be willing to share it. Remembering that Michelle was the ultimate social butterfly, I knew that she would approve, which made my decision much easier. I finally decided that I would include it at every training session that I would conduct for my company and eventually offer it up to other organizations. This gave me a wide platform in which to discuss the dangers associated with driving with distractions, considering I had ample opportunity to travel all over the country. I was already conducting OSHA training at various locations in several states, so adding one more presentation wasn't all that difficult. After the EHS conference, the first location that I would present this story, outside of North Dakota, was going to be Greeley, Colorado. By this time, I had extended the presentation to nearly forty-five minutes, and I had officially named it *Michelle's Story*.

In Greeley, the CEO of our company was visiting while I was introducing the crowd to my little sister. I was still having some anxiety issues when I told her story, and having the owner of the company sit in the audience only added to my nervousness. Putting my unsettled feelings aside, I carefully made my way through the presentation in a slow and regimented manner. In the end, it all went well, and I received the same reaction that I had received while in Bakersfield. It was becoming very clear to me that there was a genuine interest in her story, and after delivering it in Greeley, word of it was getting around. There were requests coming to me from other locations that wanted to hear it. What had started off as a request to discuss a seemingly random topic at a company conference was now beginning to become a mission for me to convey a very important message to people all over the United States.

I began sharing this message while conducting training to our newly hired employees in Minot. I was able to find a suitable spot in the training agenda and carefully crafted the narrative around our company and the oil and gas industry. I was able to find ways to tie it together with driving incidents that had occurred in our company and related policies and best practices. Slowly, the presentation began to take shape.

I was eventually able to take the presentation to several other states and cities. From North Dakota to Houston, and from Denver to locations in Utah, I was able to continue sharing the story with employees and managers everywhere I went. As rewarding as those stops were and as well as the story was received, there was one location that stands out to me the most.

It was while I was in Wheeling, West Virginia or, more

specifically, Triadelphia. My parents were living near there, in Cambridge, prior to Mom's death. Speaking here allowed me the opportunity to visit with Mom and Dad and also go to the cemetery up on the hill in Dudley and visit with Michelle. I recall hesitating to tell mom that I would be talking about Michelle's accident, because her depression was terrible, and I didn't want to make it worse. I didn't know how she would react. I was simply doing a safety audit and presenting *Michelle's Story* for the company, but she didn't want to come. I had offered a few times before for her and Dad to listen to my presentation, and I was quickly shot down. I was healing from my suffering, but Mom was drowning deeper and deeper into her despair. I didn't know how to help her, nor did I realize how deadly depression could be.

After delivering my presentation, I reflected on my time living in Ohio and all the fun times that I had experienced. I recalled the times when I would go to Charleston to visit with Michelle and Danny and all the great memories that we had all made together. I thought fondly about the time when Mitzie entered my life and when I first introduced her to Michelle. Mostly, I thought about how happy our mother seemed to be back then, back before Michelle's accident, and desperately wished we could all return to those better times. I couldn't help thinking of how much everyone's lives have changed since that stormy day in October 2005.

———

BACK HOME IN MINOT, A FRIEND AND I STARTED A small safety training business, offering various safety-related topics and OSHA training to other companies around the western part of North Dakota and eastern Montana. The business was only mildly successful and barely survived a year. We were competing with multiple safety companies that already existed, and we were late entrants into a heavily saturated market.

However, it did provide me with several more opportunities to spread the message and introduce my sister.

With every presentation, I became more comfortable discussing Michelle and her passing. I was also becoming remarkably smoother with the delivery. I still wasn't sure just how long I was going to continue sharing her story. I figured as long as people were requesting to hear it, then I wasn't going to say no. After all, it wasn't about me. I kept thinking to myself that by sharing her story, we were in some way helping at least one listener think twice and make a better decision while behind the wheel of their car.

At times, I would reflect back to that October evening and the time of her accident and wonder silently to myself if I was properly honoring her memory. Then I remembered the many times she was so helpful to others in her life. She would go out of her way to show kindness to a stranger as long as she felt they appreciated it. As I conducted these speeches, I could sense the appreciation from the various audiences, and I knew I was doing her memory justice. Often, I wished that Mike, Penny, and Denise were standing beside me as I delivered the presentation, because they were just as much a part of this journey as Michelle and I were. I love my family dearly, and I needed their support while I continued on this crusade. Mostly, I needed their constant approval and encouragement.

Every once in a while, I would reach out to my brother and sisters and let them know about the different places that I was visiting and some people that I had the privilege of talking to. We've never really been a family that openly shared our feelings with each other but, I believe that after Michelle died, we've all become much closer and truly realized that absolutely nothing in life is guaranteed.

There was something special and therapeutic with sharing her story. At times, it was as if I could almost hear her saying the words that were coming out of my mouth. Her voice was as crisp and indelible as they were when I last heard her speak. As sobering as the message about her story was, standing in front of the room and talking with different people and making incredible friends was a true joy. I started to think that I was meant to do this.

8

WHAT ABOUT DAD?

After mom's passing, our attention was quickly diverted to Dad. He hadn't been feeling very well, and because of this, he wasn't at the hospital when Mom passed away. With his breathing issues, he was only able to get out and spend some time with her on one occasion. So, after she passed away, we wanted to make sure that we all went to spend some time with Dad and make sure that he was doing alright.

When we arrived, he was quietly sitting in his chair, staring blankly at his television. I'm not even sure he was aware of what was on the screen. He looked so confused. It was almost as if he was in disbelief, and really, who could blame him? The room was dimly lit and the curtains were pulled tightly together, shielding out what little sunshine that was offered up outside. I could tell that he had been crying prior to our arrival because his eyes were watery and a bit bloodshot. A half empty tissue box was rested on an old wooden stand next to his chair. He sat in his chair with his back facing the bed where Mom had spent countless hours crying herself to sleep. It appeared to have gone untouched since she fell and was taken to the hospital. The blankets were still pulled back, as if she had just recently gotten up for the day. On the stand next to her bed, the picture of Michelle and Dean still sat propped up against her lamp. Slowly, I sat down on the bed and continued looking around the small room where Mom had spent her final days.

Penny, Denise and Mitzie tended to Dad, offering him some words of encouragement. He was now all alone and very uncertain of how to move forward. He and Mom had been married for over forty years, and he no longer had her as his companion. Throughout their marriage, he had come to depend greatly on her and she had been very loyal to him. At times, too loyal. I sometimes felt as though mom may have enabled most of Dad's perceived lack of motivation by continuously being at his beck and call. We siblings had the daunting task of helping Dad determine where he would like to spend this next chapter of his life; it was a chapter that now found him having to handle the day-to-day tasks that Mom once did for him. Our primary goal was to be there for him, but to not put ourselves in a position of having to tend to his every need. He needed to become more active and not simply give up like Mom did. We all knew that this wasn't going to be easy for Dad, but we weren't completely sure that he understood that.

We had briefly discussed having him remain in the local area by finding a small apartment in Shinglehouse, but the look on his face showed very little desire to take this route. Ronda had volunteered to help take care of him if he stayed put, but this just wasn't going to happen. When Dad didn't like something, his facial expressions fully demonstrated his dislike, and this was no exception. With his declining health, and having his happiness in mind, there was really only one option for us to seriously consider. Dad would have to move away from Shinglehouse and live with one of his children. Mike and Carrie's home was small and sat on the side of a hill with many stairs. This would be quite difficult for Dad to negotiate with the breathing issues he was dealing with. Penny and Denise both lived in smaller homes as well. Mitzie and I had the extra space, and we agreed that he should come back to North Dakota where we would be able to watch over him and get him to his medical appointments. All that was left to do was figure out the logistics involved with getting him out there. Having already done this once before, we knew that it wouldn't be an easy task, and it would involve an incredible amount of resources.

For the time being, the plan was for Dad to continue living where he was while we worked on the arrangements of moving him back out to Minot. Mike would check in on him from time to time, and Ronda helped out when needed. I was somewhat unsure about him returning to our home. He had been there before and it didn't work out. Would this time be any different? My heart hoped that it would be, but deep down inside, I knew that it probably wouldn't. Regardless of my uncertainty, he was our father, and he now needed us more than ever.

———

IT WAS LATE MARCH BY THE TIME WE WERE ABLE TO arrange his trip out to Minot. My cousin Jamie and her fiancé drove Dad and a limited amount of his personal belongings. Although it had only been a couple of months since I had last seen him, he appeared to be increasingly frail and much smaller than I had remembered. His gaunt appearance and noticeable weak walk, caused me to fear that the extremely long road trip may take a considerable toll on him and he would soon find himself in desperate need for medical care. He was only in his early seventies, but he resembled a man in his nineties. He also hadn't been taking very good care of himself and was in desperate need of a bath and a shave. It had become evident that he just wasn't doing very well at all. Living without Mom was having a serious impact on his life. I feared that he was simply giving up. It was my hope that if we made him feel as comfortable as possible, he would get back to being his normal self. I knew that he was still very upset about Mom's passing, but I didn't even consider that he may still be dealing with Michelle's death from years earlier.

We provided Dad with everything he would need. We set his room up with cable television and his own phone line. Our house was equipped with wireless internet, so he would be able to get on his computer and talk to people whenever he wanted to, and he could play his favorite games. Mitzie had set him up with a doctor to help get his health back in order, and both of us took turns shuttling him around to his various appointments. Initially, he began to show signs of improvement, and he appeared to be very happy living with us. I had hopes that his health may begin to improve as well. I empathized with my father's situation and wanted nothing more than for him to get back to being a happy, functioning member of our family. Sadly, his life began to lose balance.

As time moved forward, and spring turned to summer, Dad seemed to continue his downward slide. He continuously refused to take care of himself, and I couldn't shake that sinking feeling that I was watching my father slowly will himself to death, much like I had watched Mom do a couple years earlier. My relationship with him was also suffering, and by this point, we were barely getting along. I wanted so desperately to help him, but I didn't know how. It seemed as though we would spend the majority of time arguing with each other. Maybe we were too much alike. Who knows, but much like the last time he was in North Dakota, he wasn't content, regardless of how comfortable we made it for him.

Dealing with Dad, and his unwillingness to tend to his own basic needs, was becoming frustrating for Mitzie and me. I simply couldn't comprehend why a person would refuse to perform basic tasks, such as bathing. My lack of understanding led to many petty spats between my father and I. Sadly, I never once considered the notion that he may be dealing with extreme depression. After all, he had lost a child and, most recently, his wife of over four decades. Events, such as these, would surely have an adverse effect on a person's mental and emotional health, but for whatever reason, I just wasn't seeing this. I only saw a stubborn old man refusing to take care of himself and exercising what little control he still had over his life. I knew this couldn't go on much longer. I didn't know what the answer was, but I was fairly confident that it wasn't going to be me. I felt helpless. I was so used to being my family's protector and their rock that brought some form of stability to their somewhat chaotic lives, and now I couldn't help my father through one of the most difficult times of his life. I continued to search for other paths to take, but kept running into walls. For a brief period, we began to consider the possibility of placing Dad in a nursing home, so he could receive the ongoing care that he so desperately needed. I just couldn't bear the thought of bringing him all the way out to North Dakota only to end up putting him in a nursing home. I kept hoping that his condition and our relationship would improve, but sometimes hoping just isn't enough.

As the months rolled on, Dad quietly confided in my sister, Denise, that he no longer wanted to be in North Dakota. She had been contemplating a move to West Virginia and thought it might be better for Dad if he was closer to home and around some familiar surroundings. Dad and I still weren't getting along very well, so I agreed that he probably would be much happier in his home state. I may be happier as well. Over the next few weeks, Dad and Denise finalized their plans for getting him back to West Virginia. Denise, along with her son, Bub, were going to rent a minivan to drive Dad back. I explained to Denise how much of a toll the trip out to North Dakota had taken on him, and that she may want to break her drive up over a couple of days. I also had long conversations with her about his lack of enthusiasm and motivation to care for his most basic needs. She assured me that she would work with him on these issues, and he would be fine. She was convinced that being back where he considered home would be the best medicine for him. She was hanging on to hope.

I'm not sure how ready Dad was to make that long trip, but ready or not, he was going to make it. I was amazed to see that he had started showing signs of life once he knew he was leaving. He packed some small things and began to move around a bit more than I had seen him previously. His sudden burst of energy nearly broke my heart. Was it me? I know we weren't getting along very well. We would often argue about the way he was caring for himself, or the lack thereof, but he seemed to be much more active than he had been since arriving in Minot. Clearly, he was excited about leaving. I decided that I would let him get settled into the small house that Denise had rented for them, and then I would call him and attempt to talk through our issues.

As the time was nearing for Denise and Bub to come out, Mitzie and I began purchasing some odds and ends for them to take back for their home. We couldn't allow Dad to go all the way back to West Virginia without sending him off with some gifts. We also wanted to make sure Denise had enough supplies to prepare meals for her and Dad. This would also provide me with the opportunity to spend a little time with my twin sister and nephew. I hadn't seen Bub since Michelle's funeral and was looking forward to seeing him.

9

ANOTHER TRAGEDY HITS HOME

Paul III, better known as Bub, was Denise and Junior's youngest of the three children they had together. Bub wasn't like his older sisters. There was something a little different about him. He reminded me a lot of Mike's son, Cameron. While growing up, neither seemed to have a care in the world, and they were very content being outside and playing as rough as they could. Even at a young age, Bub was a very tough kid. He was no stranger to receiving bumps and bruises. From time to time, he would make his way back into the house in need of a band-aid or two. As a small child, he had incredible strength, and he would often be seen carrying some heavy items, such as logs or bricks.

Much like his Aunt Michelle used to do, Bub would antagonize his sisters, and for the better part, get away with it. Being the youngest kid and the only son, his antics were often overlooked, and his sisters, Brandie and Heather would simply have to learn how to deal with it. They had a pretty good person in their corner to teach them how to do that, because Denise learned that same lesson as a child.

Bub was also an early learner. He seemed to walk at a much

younger age than other children. He picked up on remedial tasks sooner than one might expect a child to do. He was around three years old, I believe, when he first learned to completely balance a bicycle without training wheels. Many of the people around him were left in amazement. Not only could he balance the bike and maneuver it around, but he remained seated the entire time, whether he was peddling up a hill or coasting down the other side. His leg strength was truly amazing. I used to comment that he was going to become a football player when he got older.

Bub was always a momma's boy. As much as his dad wanted him to have similar interests as he did, such as hunting or fishing, Bub was more interested in going wherever Denise went and hanging out with her. He worshiped the ground his mother walked on, but she wasn't immune to his antagonistic ways. At times, he would push her buttons much like his sisters, and when she got frustrated, he would run away laughing. Well, at least until she caught up with him. A child with his abundance of energy and mischievous nature often found himself sitting in the corner, getting a spanking, or going to bed early. There were times when Denise and Junior wondered just how they were going to find the energy to keep up with their youngest cub.

Bub was the apple of his grandfather's eye. Junior's father, Paul Sr., really took to Bub. Of course, he was the last male to carry on their family name. If Bub thought he could get away with whatever he wanted to at home, this seemed to be extenuated when he was at his grandparents' place. This further proved to drive Brandie and Heather crazy. Maybe it was because he was the youngest child, or maybe it was because he was the only son. Whatever the reason, Bub seemed to be treated a bit differently than the girls and took full advantage of that.

Growing up, Bub learned that if he wanted something, he would have to work for it. This was a trait that was instilled in him from an early age. He was a very hard worker throughout his teenage years. It wasn't uncommon to see him helping his father or grandfather performing rather strenuous labor around their respective homesteads. As his school years came to an end, he was able to secure a job at a local lumber mill, not far from his grandparents' home. This was the same mill that Junior's brother and I both worked at many years earlier. Although I personally believe he would have excelled in college, that was something that just wasn't in his plans. Bub was a blue-collar sort of young man, and he was most content performing hard, manual labor daily. He was quite good at it.

As hard as Bub worked, he also played equally hard. Consuming beer and weekend hangouts with friends were as much a part of the local fabric as anything else. During the summer months, you could drive down the endless miles of country roads and see numerous bonfires. Each had a large crowd of participants in their own respective hillbilly rituals. During my time living in southeastern Ohio, I was a guest at many of these gatherings and certainly consumed my fair share of adult beverages. I rarely turned down an opportunity to attend one of these events, and Denise and Junior were no strangers at throwing these festive galas. Many of them were held at their residence. Working hard and enjoying the fruits of his labor wasn't necessarily a learned behavior for Bub; this was simply a rite of passage for him and his sisters.

I lost track of Bub after Mitzie and I moved to North Dakota, but I would often ask Denise how he and his sisters were doing. I spent a great deal of time around those kids when they were younger, and they always had a special place in my heart. Don't get me wrong, I love all my nieces and nephews a great deal, but there just seemed to be a little extra something about those three. I was able to continue to watch them all grow through the advancements of social media and periodic visits back east. The girls were much quicker about using the computer to share their personal experiences than Bub. This made keeping up with him a bit more difficult, especially since I was living so far away. It didn't help that when Bub became a teenager, Denise and Junior separated and went their own ways.

As he became more comfortable using the computer, he began to share things, such as pictures of his girlfriend and stories about certain events occurring in his life. Of course, he would also share pictures and stories of some next-generation parties and gatherings that he and his friends attended. He seemed to be enjoying life and doing what nearly every young man had done before him on nearly every weekend. It wasn't uncommon to see him with one arm around a friend of his and a cold beer in the opposite hand. His young life was taking shape, and he was following his chosen path with vigor and enthusiasm.

Whenever his mother needed something done, Bub was always quick to accommodate her. So, it came as no surprise to me that he volunteered to accompany Denise on her journey out to Minot to transport Dad back to West Virginia. I couldn't wait to see him when she told me that he was coming out with her. I wanted to catch up with him and find out how things were going for him. Mainly, I just wanted to see just how much that little boy I remembered had grown. I was also happy to know that Denise and dad had him along as a protector during their long drive. I would have been a nervous wreck if it was just those two. With all of dad's health issues, she would have been forced to drive the entire time. Having Bub with her brought me peace of mind.

When Denise and Bub finally arrived at our house, I was amazed at just how large he was. He easily stood six foot three, inches and weighed approximately two-hundred and thirty pounds. He didn't have much fat on hisself; he was solid muscle.

"Man, you've gotten big," I said. "If anyone ever gives me trouble, I'm gonna stand behind you." Of course, I was just kidding, but he had gone from a small boy to a very large young man.

Bub chuckled a bit and quietly said, "Yeah, I suppose."

His demeanor didn't seem to fit his overall appearance and

size. I really expected him to be loud and very outgoing, but he proved to be quite the opposite. Although his voice was deep, his tone was soft, and he appeared to be somewhat shy. Perhaps it was because he hadn't seen Mitzie or I for a few years. Who knows? The way he carried himself led me to believe that he was a very genuine young man. A gentle giant, I guess you could say.

Denise made her way into Dad's room to let him know that they had arrived. I could hear her and Dad talking and laughing while I visited with Bub in the kitchen. After a few minutes, Denise joined us in the living room and slowly sipped at her cup of coffee that Mitzie had made for her. She looked incredibly tired and appeared to need some sleep. Mitzie was showing her some items that we had picked up at our local Walmart for her and Dad to take back to their new home.

After some time, Denise decided she wanted to get ready for bed and made her way to the bedroom that Mitzie had prepared for her. Bub wanted to sit up for a while and have a couple of beers, but I wasn't able to stay up very long with him because I had to work the following day. I kept thinking to myself that I should have taken some vacation time so I could spend more time with him and Denise while they were in. Denise had mentioned that they would be leaving in a couple days in order to give us plenty of time to get Dad's things together and spend some quality time with both of them.

On the morning they were scheduled to leave, I asked Denise if she was going to be okay with taking care of Dad. She knew of the struggles that Mitzie and I had dealt with during his stay at our home, and she could sense my concerns.

"He's going to be fine," she said. I knew she was trying to put my mind at ease, but she wasn't all that convincing with that statement. I had no choice now but to trust that everything would work out and she would be able to care for Dad and get him to help care for himself.

I never got to see them off on the morning that they left

Minot. I was at work when they began their trip to West Virginia. I asked Denise and Bub to stay in touch throughout their journey and to let me know when they arrived in Clarksburg. I was a bit saddened when I got home from work to see Dad's room empty. I don't even remember saying goodbye to him the night before. I punished myself for not being very nice to him while he was here. After all, there had to be a reason he didn't want to live with me, and in my mind, it was me. Shaking my head, I turned and walked out of his room, slowly closing the door behind me.

———

I WASN'T AT ALL PREPARED FOR THE PHONE CALL THAT I received from Dad that late November evening. I should have been prepared, I mean, after all, I had had plenty of experience getting these heartbreaking phone calls from him. When I heard Dad's voice on the other end, I braced myself for the impending bad news that typically accompanied his calls.

"Dennis?" he asked. He had that all-to-familiar sound in his voice that I had heard before when Mom ended up in the hospital. It was almost as if he didn't want to call me, but he felt some sort of obligation to do so I could hear Denise crying in the background, which caused my mind to scramble. I didn't know what had occurred, but I knew that whatever it was, it wasn't going to be good. That very same thought had crossed my mind far too many times in the past, and now, I was once again preparing myself to learn some more bad news.

"Yeah, what's up Dad?" I responded.

"Bub was in a car wreck and died." Those words penetrated my brain, sending shock waves through my entire body. Dad wasn't one to mince words and usually said it like it was. I remember having to sit down as I tried to make sense of this bit of information. "Here, Denise wants to talk to ya," he said, trying to get off the phone.

There was a long pause as I waited for someone, anyone, to begin talking again. I was quietly relaxing in my recliner watching television, and suddenly another piece of my world would be gone forever. I was so confused. I was now at the edge of my seat and intently listening to the background noises in my phone when the silence was suddenly broken by my sister; she frantically tried to explain to me what had happened.

"I lost my baby, Dennis!" she screamed into the phone. She must have repeated that same sentence a dozen times while talking to me. I needed to find out what had happened, but she was crying so hard that I was unable to gain her attention long enough to get a clear response out of her. I asked for her to give the phone back to Dad or to someone who would have the capacity to communicate a bit more clearly. I knew she just needed to talk, but I also knew she needed to gather herself as much as she could and calm down a bit, if that was even possible at this point.

Brandie took over the phone call and explained to me that Bub was in a car accident. He rolled his vehicle on a curve and was ejected, dying at the scene. I couldn't believe what I was hearing.

Oh, dear Lord. Not again. I thought to myself. It was suddenly becoming crystal clear to me that much like Michelle a little over a decade earlier, my nephew had lost his life in a completely preventable car accident. I just needed to hear the details that were being relayed to me in bits and pieces, and then I needed to put them together in my mind to help make sense of yet another family tragedy. *How could this happen again?* I thought.

My mind was suddenly overwhelmed by memories of Michelle's death and the seemingly irreversible impact it had on our mother. Denise now found herself in that very same situation. She had lost a child, and by the sounds echoing through my phone, her personal struggle was just beginning. I wished I could be there for her, to do something, anything.

"Oh Denise," I mumbled under my breath. "I'm so sorry."

I couldn't dismiss the thoughts of how Mom's life had significantly changed, and I knew that Denise was in for a long, emotional ride that far too many parents across this country have taken but shouldn't have had to. I had watched Mom slowly fade away for a decade, not able to do anything about it until, one day in a northern Pennsylvania hospital, her life had finally come to an end. As bad as I was hurting at the sudden, tragic loss of Bub, my heart was aching for my twin sister and her two daughters.

I could clearly remember how devastated Denise was when Michelle had died, and how it had taken her years to recover from it and begin healing. Surely this would be far too much for her to handle this time. It had been less than a year since Mom had passed away, and we were still mourning. She would certainly need somebody to be with her for a while, especially as she was about to hit the highways and travel to Ohio. She had Penny that she could lean on, but what she really needed was Brandie and Heather, and they needed her just as much.

After ending my phone call, I once again sat quietly in my recliner and wiped away some tears that I had grown far too accustomed to shedding. I kept thinking about Bub through the various stages of his life, and I wondered how we had gotten to this point. How did we lose another family member in a vehicle accident? He was on an old country road that he had traveled hundreds of times before. Over a short period, some details surrounding his accident started coming out. I learned that Bub was leaving one of those weekend parties, that all of us had attended at one time or another in our lives. He missed a turn and rolled his vehicle. He had only driven a couple hundred yards down the road before losing control of his car and rolling it into a field. He was so close that those still at the party had heard the accident and ran down to the scene to assess the damage. One of those party-goers was Bub's older sister, Heather. Just as Penny had done years earlier, Heather bore witness to her sibling's fatality.

I remember thinking that my family may be cursed in some way. How else do you begin to explain two precious souls snatched away while in the prime of their lives? Two lives gone because of vehicle accidents. This was unfathomable to me. I've never known another family that has experienced the loss of two relatives, few years apart, in a similar manner. As I continued to think about this recent event, I began to go from intense sadness to a bit of anger. I couldn't understand why the other party-goers would allow him to drive his car away after an evening of consuming alcohol.

"Why did they let him drive?" I said out loud. "Why didn't someone get his keys?"

"You can't go there, Dennis," Mitzie chimed in. "He's a grownup and responsible for himself."

Mitzie always had a way of being the voice of sound reasoning. She was always able to get me to see the bigger picture and not simply focus on the event alone. This is the trait that I adored most about her. Through all these trying times in my life, she was always able to keep me grounded and focused. She was well aware that my family leaned on me for support and wasn't going to allow me to get lost in the details. Bub was gone, and there wasn't anything I could do about it. I needed to concentrate on Denise and give her as much emotional support as I possibly could. She was my priority; trying to investigate the root cause of a vehicle accident was not.

————

ONCE DENISE HAD FINALLY MADE HER WAY TO OHIO for Bub's funeral, I knew that she was going to experience the various levels of grief that usually accompany the loss of a loved one, especially a child. I was just hoping that she wouldn't experience all of those levels at one time when she arrived at the funeral. She could, at times, be somewhat unpredictable, and she was known to express her sadness in loud and animated ways. It made me feel better knowing that she would have Heather and Brandie with her through this process. I was also comforted to know that Mike and Penny were both going to be there. As sad as it was, we all had experience with this, having gone through this process with Mom. Now, we all had to help Denise get through this as well.

I was unable to travel to Ohio for Bub's funeral. I depended on Mike and Penny to provide me with the details of how the day had gone. From all accounts, the funeral went as well as could be expected. Junior and Denise, who rarely agreed on anything since they had separated years earlier, stood side by side and said goodbye to their son. They both had a long road ahead of them and would each travel their own in very different ways. Denise would soon make her way back down to North Carolina, but she was in no condition to care for Dad. For a very long time, she was barely able to take care of herself. Heather continued to reside in Marietta, Ohio, and Brandie returned to her residence in North Carolina with her mother. Much like with Michelle, everyone soon realized that the sun would come up tomorrow, and life would painfully have to go on.

For me, I called each of my children and had pointed conversations about driving while under the influence or with other equally dangerous distractions. Above all, I didn't want to see this happen for a third time during my lifetime. Our family tree was now missing some precious leaves. Leaves that were once vibrant and alive had now left the tree and softly floated away in the breeze, leaving behind empty spots on the branches.

10

THE TIES THAT BIND

I wasn't all that surprised when Penny called to tell me that Dad was admitted to the hospital with breathing issues. Over the years, I had become fairly familiar with his difficulties with breathing. He had been experiencing problems for quite some time, mainly because he had always been a smoker. His smoking dates back to his teen years when he would sneak away to a quiet place to enjoy a freshly rolled menthol cigarette. He was originally diagnosed with COPD a while back due to breathing in coal dust for years while growing up in West Virginia. Over time, this had caused his breathing to become more labored and difficult, and the smoking certainly didn't help. This wasn't his first trip to the hospital, so I figured the medical staff would give him some medications and a steady supply of oxygen and send him on his way in a day or two. That's how it usually went when he went to the hospital. Then Penny went into greater detail.

"So, the doctors told us that his breathing isn't going to get any better," she said. Much like Dad, Penny was one to always say it like it is and not mince words. She would deal with the emotions later. I always appreciated that about her. Normally, she would sound upbeat and positive when discussing matters such as these, but this time she had a quiet and serious tone. We've been down this road before, and it gave me an uneasy feeling listening to her.

"Are they going to let him come home?" I asked. What I had thought was going to be a simple hospital visit, to correct a shortness of breath issue, had suddenly turned into much more. This was clearly very serious. "What else are they saying?" I asked.

"They're going to send him to a nursing home for a little while when he is discharged, so they can continue to treat him," Penny added. "He's probably not going to ever be able to live on his own."

I just wanted to talk to him. I wanted to hear his voice and know for myself that he was okay. Listening to Penny's choice of words allowed me to read between the lines. If his breathing was never going to improve, then how much time would he have left? What would his quality of life be like once he was released from the nursing home?

"How's he doing now? I asked.

"He seems to be okay," Penny responded. "He's been joking around with the nurses. They're getting ready to clean him up, so I'm going to get out of here till tomorrow."

"Alright," I reluctantly said. "Keep me updated, please."

After our phone call ended, I sat back and found myself, once again, deeply concerned for a family member. I knew Dad's health wasn't all that good, and I really should have expected to hear this news, but as prepared as you think you are, you're really never ready to hear news like this.

As I continued to worry about Dad, my mind wandered back in time to some of our better moments. I reminisced about my time in the military, and how dad would see to it that I arrived safely at each of my duty stations by personally driving me there.

Back in the day, he really enjoyed driving and would often travel to many places. Maybe this is where Michelle acquired her love of the highway. Dad was a very good driver. I always thought that he would have been a great truck driver. He was the only person that I completely trusted to drive while I slept.

These trips, traveling to and from military installations, provided us with some much- needed father-son time. Sadly, these moments didn't last forever. As I grew older, got married, and began my own family, we rarely got along. However, as a young man going from base to base, I depended on him greatly. In some ways, I think he appreciated that. Even when we would argue and not see eye to eye, I still missed all the times that we had spent on the road. He was a large part of my military career.

The following morning, I asked Penny if dad was feeling well enough to talk. I had spent the better part of the evening thinking about him and really wanted to hear his voice. I didn't know what I was going to say to him. For years, our stubbornness had gotten the best of us, and for whatever reason, I found it best to just not talk to him.

"Hey Dad, how ya doing?" I asked, then I sat quietly and waited for his response. We hadn't talked to each other since he called to tell us about Bub. *Did he even want to talk to me?* I thought to myself.

"Doing good," he said in his unique southern twang. His voice was very upbeat, and he sounded happy to hear from me. "When I get out of here, Penny's gonna help me get my own place," he continued. He sounded like a new man. His sentences were broken with forced deep breaths as he talked. "How are you all doing?" he asked.

"We're doing well, Dad." I could almost feel myself beginning to choke up as I listened to him talk. I could clearly hear him struggle with each word. Suddenly, all the issues that he and I had gone through in the past meant nothing to me. I just wanted to reach out and give him a hug. The guilt for all the wasted time weighed heavily on my heart. "I think you would do well in your own place," I added, even though I remembered Penny saying that he wouldn't be able to live by himself. I just let him talk while I listened and smiled.

Dad wasn't able to stay on the phone for very long because he was having a hard time catching his breath, but I promised him that I would call him again soon. For the first time in a long time, I truly meant it.

Dad continued improving over the next couple of weeks on some sort of physical therapy regiment. I'm not sure what all it consisted of, but he never complained about having to do it when I would talk with him. The doctors put him on a continuous supply of oxygen, and when he eventually returned home, wherever that would be, he would have tanks there as well. Aside from his troubled breathing, the doctors also had some concern over an aneurism located near his kidneys. He had had a medical issue in the past regarding an aneurism that nearly took his life. This bit of news really made me nervous. Penny explained that they wouldn't be able to surgically remove it until they could stabilize his breathing. Through it all, he remained positive and seemed to look forward to whatever life was going to bring his way.

A day or so after he began physical therapy, Dad was moved to the nursing home to continue his rehabilitation. With everything considered, he seemed to enjoy the nursing home. He quickly befriended an older gentleman, and he began sharing fishing tales and stories of his childhood in West Virginia. As much as I wished he didn't have to be in a nursing home, this appeared to be an ideal place for him, at least for a little while. Our main goal was for him to be able to function well enough to eventually make it back home where he could truly be comfortable. Remarkably, it had now been several weeks since he was first admitted to the hospital and we had yet to hear him complain.

———

A COUPLE OF WEEKS LATER, PENNY FOUND DAD A SMALL but nice trailer to live in. This was the first time in a very long time that he had a place that he could call his own. Penny checked in on him several times each day to make sure he was doing okay. She would send the rest of us periodic updates and pictures of him relaxing on his porch or preparing his own dinner. I was very happy that he was doing well, even though he had to wander around with a long clear hose connecting him to his oxygen supply.

He sounded and looked so much better than I had remembered since Mom's passing. He finally seemed happy and content. I couldn't remember the last time I had seen him smile or laugh so much. Perhaps he was finally getting past the grief of losing so many people in his life. Maybe he was finally freeing himself from whatever guilt he had spent years holding onto. I didn't care what the reason was. I was just glad he had finally turned the page and was going to make the most of whatever time he had left.

Not long after moving into the trailer and getting comfortable with his new digs, Dad had a relapse, and he soon found himself back in the hospital. Talking with Penny, he had apparently been unable to catch his breath, even with the oxygen supply. Maybe the doctors were right. Maybe he would never be able to live on his own. Even though Penny and Ed checked on him daily, sometimes several times a day, they couldn't be there all the time. If he was going to live outside a nursing home, he would need constant care.

A few days after his return to the hospital, Dad, once again, found himself back in the nursing home rehabilitating. Realizing that Dad shouldn't be alone any longer, Penny's son, Chris, offered to share a residence with him. Dad's current trailer was only a one-bedroom place so, Penny searched for another one, and soon found one not far from his previous trailer. This one was located near a small lake that was surrounded by a forest full of tall pines. When Penny explained all of this to Dad, he was excited to see his new home, and he was looking forward to sharing it with Chris.

This trip to the hospital was much different than the previous one. This time, the doctors really didn't want him to return to living away from medical care, so they placed Dad in the care of hospice before they would allow him to return home.

————

PENNY AND CHRIS WERE ABLE TO COMPLETELY MOVE Dad's things into the new trailer in a single day. When Dad finally arrived, he sat on the couch and looked around in amazement.

"Your mom would have loved this place," he said.

He was also pleased with the view that he had. Dad was always a person who enjoyed nature, so having all the pines and the lake within his immediate view brought him joy. Penny set his bedroom up with everything he would need, but he never slept a night in it. Dad was quite content simply sleeping on his couch with the television remote, an ashtray, and a glass of soda within arm's reach. Chris took the bedroom located at the other end of the trailer, adjoining the kitchen. It was September when they moved into their new home, so the prominent Carolina heat was still in full force. His comfort and safety were the top priority for Penny and Chris. Making sure the air conditioning was in perfect working order was paramount. Fortunately, Penny's husband, Ed, was an air conditioning technician.

Representatives from Pruitt Hospice had a hospital bed delivered for Dad. They placed the bed in the living room and positioned it so he could look out the window and have a constant view of the lake. Still, it would be a few days before Dad would begin actually sleeping in his new bed. I'm not sure why he initially refused to sleep in the hospital bed. I think that he may have been tired of being in one. I also believe that when he saw the bed, along with the hospice nurses, he realized that they were now preparing him for his final days. That had to be very frightening for him. After some coaxing from Penny and Chris, Dad finally relented and began sleeping in the hospital bed.

As fall turned into winter, Dad's mobility was increasingly limited. He lost his strength and was fully dependent on Penny and Chris. The hospice nurses prepared everyone for the various stages that patients typically encounter while in hospice care. I'm not sure if Dad truly understood what hospice was. I think he was under the impression that the nurses coming to his home were there simply to check on his medications, order oxygen refills, and work with his mobility. He and Chris were doing well, and for all intents and purposes, they made really good roommates. The more restricted Dad became, the more Chris was doing for him.

There were a few nurses that came by to work with Dad. Mamie and Lover were his favorites. He talked often about how well they treated him. In fact, he would mention them so much when we talked on the phone, that you would think that they were close relatives. Penny often said that they enjoyed spending time with him as well. That didn't really surprise me because Dad had always been able to get along well with relative strangers.

I tried to call and talk with Dad, at least once every week, but I would call more often when I was able to. I was at a point in my life where I really liked having conversations with him. Undoubtedly, our conversation would ultimately turn into discussions about football, which was a passion of both of ours. Dad loved to talk about his favorite team, the Seattle Seahawks. He would tell me how they were going to win another Super

Bowl. I'm not sure how he ever became a fan of a team that plays on the west coast, but since my childhood, I had always remembered him being a Seattle fan.

I really didn't care what we talked about just as long as we kept talking. I'm not sure what Penny did, but she was able to do with dad what none of us ever could. He seemed to make a complete transformation when she got involved in his care. He went from a difficult and stubborn individual to a person that laughed often and never seemed to complain about his current situation. Perhaps, he was finally resigning himself to the fact that he was on limited time, and just wanted to enjoy all of it. Each time we would hang up, I had a smile on my face and was looking forward to our next conversation. Dad and I had certainly rounded a corner in our relationship. Much like the coastal winds that push the storm clouds away to clear the sky and allow the sun to make its appearance, Dad and I were able to clear the air between us, put our differences aside, and simply enjoy each other's company. For the first time in a very long time, I fully realized just how important having my father in my life was, and I didn't want to waste another minute of whatever precious time we had left.

———

IT WAS MARCH WHEN PENNY BEGAN INDICATING THAT his condition was quickly deteriorating. There were stages to the hospice process, as we had previously learned. It was clear that he was now moving through them. One afternoon, Penny called me to update me on his condition. I looked forward to these updates, but this one came with a particular request. Possibly sensing that he was running short on time, Dad had made a comment to Penny about how nice it would be to have all the kids together for a dinner. Penny knew that it was simply time to get everyone together to come see him while we still could.

"Hey, how's it going?" I asked.

"If, at all possible, ya'll need to come out here and see Dad," Penny said, sounding more like a demand than a request. I could sense some urgency in her voice. "This may be the last chance you'll have."

"Alright," I said. "I'll have Mitzie start looking at some flights."

Penny had decided that she would wait until I made my travel arrangements before she let Mike and Denise know about our plans to have a make-shift Easter dinner with Dad. I asked her to keep it a secret from Dad unless his condition became much worse. I wanted to surprise him with a visit. She was able to keep it quiet for a while, but Dad soon figured out what was going on, and he looked forward to everyone's arrival. Mitzie wouldn't be able to make the trip out, but she secured flights for Nicky and I for mid-April.

———

NICKY AND I LANDED IN CHARLOTTE, AND AFTER securing our rental car, we began our drive to Spring Lake to see Penny, Ed, Chris, and most importantly, Dad. I thought of the upcoming days, spending time visiting with family, and enjoying each other's company. I couldn't wait to see Dad, but I was a bit nervous as to what I would see when I got there. The last photo I had was of him. He was sitting on his deck, holding his arms in the air, as if he was showing everyone that he was free from whatever had been holding him down. I loved that picture. No matter how many more were taken of him, that would be the one that I would display on my mantle next to Mom's picture.

After a couple hour's drive, we pulled into Dad's driveway and was met outside by Penny. I reached out and gave her a hug, and we made our way into Dad's trailer. I walked through the front door and saw Dad quietly sleeping on his hospital bed. I stared down at him. He looked so frail and gaunt. He was never a big person and had always been thin, but he had lost even more weight since I last saw him.

"Hey Dad," I quietly said, not wanting to disturb him, but selfishly hoping he would wake up. Right on cue, his eyes slowly opened, and he turned his head slightly to look up at me. With a tired smile, he reached his hand out and tapped me on the arm. I bent down and gave him the hug that I had long wanted to give him. "How have you been?" I asked.

"Good," he softly said, while shaking his head. Looking around the room, he noticed Nicky standing near us and smiled even bigger. "Well hello, Nicky," he said.

Nicky had always been a quiet kid and somewhat reserved, but he walked over and stood next to me beside Dad's bed, answering his question. "I'm good."

A short time later, Denise had arrived, followed soon after by our half-sister, Sherry, and her family. They each went to Dad's bedside to let him know that they had made it in. As people continued flooding into the living room, Dad smiled and stared in disbelief. Although Penny had mentioned that he knew we were coming in, I honestly think he may have forgotten about it.

"Wow, look at everyone," he said.

Mike hadn't yet made it in because he was traveling up from Tennessee in his semi. He was coming off the road and was going to spend a few days with all of us. I had told him to give me a call when he got into town, and I would go meet him. As I watched Dad talking and laughing with everyone, I couldn't help but wonder if he fully understood why so many of his loved ones were randomly showing up in April to come and spend time with him. Looking at his face, he seemed to be completely surprised. I wonder if he even remembered his simple request that he had shared with Penny. Because of his declining health, we were all coming eventually anyway, but his previous wish had certainly moved our visits along a little quicker.

About a half hour later, I received a call from Mike, letting me know that he had arrived in Spring Lake. I met him a couple miles down the road, where he found a lot to drop his trailer off for a couple days. I had him follow me to Penny and Ed's home, where he parked his vehicle. Once he had his truck parked and shut down, he climbed into my rental vehicle, and we made our way back over to Dad's place.

After everyone spent some time visiting with Dad, we all gathered around a small fire pit out front and caught up with each other. Dad's stamina didn't allow him to stay awake for long periods of time, so we left him alone and let him get his rest. We would all have plenty of time to catch up with him later. Penny and I had planned on having a memorable Easter dinner with Dad, so we began making our shopping list and creating our menu. I didn't care what the cost was; I was going to make sure that our feast with Dad was splendid. I wanted everyone to be happy and have a really good time. We all knew that Dad didn't have much time left, but we weren't going to sulk and be sad around him. We were going to celebrate our belated Easter dinner.

The next morning, Nicky and I drove over to Dad's, beginning our special day with him. We walked in, and he was already awake and joking around with everyone. He was looking at an older laptop of Nicky's that we had brought out for him. Dad always liked playing games on the computer, but theirs was a desktop and he couldn't get himself over to a desk to enjoy it any longer. I walked over to his bedside and stood beside him. Leaning over, I gave him a hug and helped prop his pillow up under him a bit.

"How you doing today, Dad?" I asked.

"I feel good," he responded. "Do you smell all that good cooking out there?" he continued. It was early, but Denise had prepared coffee for everyone, and she was already beginning to cook the ham for dinner later on. Between her and Penny, they were going to prepare all the food.

"Yeah, I could smell it when I got out of the van," I said. He was clearly very excited and was going to enjoy every minute of this day. I took myself into the kitchen to get a hot cup of coffee and visit with Denise for a couple of minutes. She was in the process of cutting up potatoes.

"Need some help peeling these?"

"No, I've got this," she said. Denise has spent nearly her entire adult life in the restaurant business, and she was a very good cook. There wasn't much that she didn't know how to prepare. We were joined a couple minutes later by Chris and then Mike. I asked Chris if he wanted to get out for a while and run around with Mike, Nicky, and me. With all the time that he had been spending helping to care for Dad, he rarely had any time to sneak away and relax. Besides, Dad was visiting with the girls and likely wouldn't miss us.

"We'll be back in a little bit," I told Denise. "You need anything while we're out?"

"No, I'm good," she said.

After letting Dad know that we were leaving for a while, the four of us ventured out for a couple hours. I could tell that Chris was a little worn out from taking care of Dad and enjoyed being able to get away and spend some time with us. We drove to a local grocery store to pick up a few things that we had forgotten earlier, then we stopped at a small pawn shop to see if we were able to find any good deals.

After a couple of hours, we made our way back to Dad's to get ready for our family dinner and continue our impromptu family reunion. I noticed that Dad was sleeping, so I found a place to sit and made myself comfortable. Watching my father rest peacefully forced my mind to drift to a much simpler time. I reminisced on some of our childhood and conjured up some fond memories. I thought about the time that Mike and I taught Michelle how to ride a bicycle by pushing her down the hill in Farmington. I thought of the rustic old cabin that was barely livable in Beverly, Ohio. I thought back on playing football in high school and recalled the times I would look into the bleachers and find my father bundled in a light jacket, attempting to stay warm on a chilly fall evening; he would sit alone intently watching his oldest son.

With the soft, sudden whine of the front door, I noticed Penny and Sherry making their way to the kitchen to help put the final touches on the dinner. I watched as Penny and Sherry laughed while pulling items from the refrigerator and placing them on the table. I then shifted my attention toward Denise, who was still standing in front of the stove, slowly stirring the contents that she had placed in the small, black pot moments earlier. Standing with her back to me, I couldn't help but notice just how much Denise reminded me of our mother. She stood quietly watching the steam rolling up from the heated pot in front of her. It brought back cherished memories of the many times I watched Mom prepare meals for all of us.

Although she wasn't saying anything, her body language let us all know that she was heavy with sadness. We all felt that this may well be the final time we would all have to sit together and enjoy a meal with our ailing father. In many ways, I watched my twin sister turn into Mom right before my eyes. In reality, I had been watching her for a while. Much like mom, Denise suffered with the painful loss of her youngest child. I thought about the many times when I was unable to reach her on the phone. She would call me back, apologize, and let me know that she was sleeping. Mom used to sleep, a lot. It wasn't lost on me that Denise also openly wore her depression. My heart ached for my sister. But just like my mother, I felt helpless. I didn't know how to help Mom through her inner battles, and I struggled to know how to help Denise.

Mike and Ed joined me in the living room. I thought about a

time when we didn't have the best clothes or live in the nicest houses, but we always seemed to laugh. Because we moved around a lot, we never had many friends, but we always had each other. We never had any material wealth, but I now realize that we were rich beyond belief.

After a prayer from Ed, we enjoyed our abundant family feast. The dinner was incredible and everyone ate until they were nearly busting at the seams. We sat around in the living room and shared stories with Dad. As enjoyable and festive as the day had been, there were a few people missing. Penny mentioned that Mom and Michelle would have loved this small gathering. The smile never left Dad's face, even when he was noticeably tired. We decided to let Dad get some sleep, and we went outside to sit around a fire pit to continue our walk down memory lane. It was an awesome day, and I was so glad that Nicky and I were able to make it out to be a part of it. I was especially happy that we were able to mend our fences and finally enjoy each other's company.

On the day that Nicky and I were scheduled to drive back to Charlotte, we woke up early, packed the rental van, and drove to Dad's to spend the morning with him before we had to leave. It had truly been a great visit, and I wasn't ready to leave. I wanted to take full advantage of every last minute I had with him.

When we arrived, he was eating his breakfast, consisting of a small pile of scrambled eggs, two slices of toast with jelly, some leftover ham from the previous day, and his usual cup of coffee.

"Are you hungry?" he asked.

I politely passed on the offer for breakfast, explaining that we had grabbed some breakfast at McDonalds before coming over. We engaged in small talk, but mostly I listened to his voice. After a couple of hours, it was time for us to leave. I bent down and gave Dad a hug and a kiss on his forehead.

"I love you, Dad."

"I love you too, son," he said. "Thanks for coming out, and tell Mitzie and the boys I said hi."

"I sure will," I added.

Before getting into the vehicle, I turned around and looked back at the front door. "See ya later, Dad," I quietly said to myself.

We pulled out of the driveway, drove down the bumpy dirt road, and turned right on to an adjoining avenue that would lead us out of the neighborhood. The further away we got, the more I wanted to turn around and go back so I could spend some more time with him. Tears welled up in the corners of my eyes. I knew that when I left Dad's trailer, that would likely be the final time I would see him. Nicky quietly asked me, *"Are you okay, Dad?"*

I couldn't be better, I thought to myself.

————

ONE WEEK AFTER LEAVING SPRING LAKE, ON APRIL 28TH, Penny called to let us know that Dad had passed away peacefully in his bed. She mentioned that when he died, his head was facing a picture of mom and him. It was as if he was letting her know that his pain and suffering was now over and he would be with her. I thanked Penny and Chris for everything they had done for Dad. I reminded them that they were able to do something that nobody else had ever been able to. They brought Dad comfort and happiness during the final year of his life.

Although my heart was broken, and the tears flowed freely, I was content knowing that his final wish was fulfilled. He had mentioned that he wanted to have dinner with his children, and he got so much more. We all did. I sat down in my recliner, once again thinking back on our travels to and from the military bases, I quietly thought to myself, *Rest easy, Dad.*

CHAPTER 11: THE JOURNEY CONTINUES- MICHELLE'S Story Today

Through all the loss my family has experienced and in an effort to get her very important message to as many listeners as possible, I remained steadfast and continued sharing Michelle's story. What began as an exercise in healing and acceptance has now become a calling in my life. Her story has grown, both in size and in scope because of the events that have transpired since her accident.

Looking back on that rain-soaked highway, near the coast of North Carolina, in October 2005, it truly amazes me how one single event, one tragic death, could have such a rippling effect through one family. Since her accident, our family has lost a mother, a father, and a nephew, and for my sister Denise, a son. Should one family suffer so much loss in such a short period of time? That's a question that probably doesn't have an answer. Besides, who am I to question God's will?

For as much as her story has evolved, and of all the people that I talk about when sharing it, there was one person noticeably absent from my presentations. I realized that I don't talk much about Dad when I do the presentation. I do talk about Mom and the struggles and personal torment that she experienced for a ten-year period following Michelle's death. I've given this considerable thought and simply cannot explain why I continue failing to include my father when I speak. After all, he lost just as much as Mom. The pain he felt had to be much like hers. So why wouldn't I discuss him when I share this story? Maybe it's because he didn't outwardly show his grief, or perhaps it's because deep down inside, I knew that he would be very uncomfortable with me talking about him to a group of perfect strangers. Who knows? Whatever the reason, Michelle's story has evolved from discussing a terrible car accident and death of a beautiful young woman to a story about an accident that would test the emotional strength of a somewhat fractured family.

Over the years, each of my family members has dealt with her death in their own unique way. Some openly displayed their grief and sadness, while others were not so transparent. For me, I decided for a long time to not talk about it. It wasn't until I began traveling and doing my presentations that I discovered the ability and willingness to discuss how her car accident affected me. I didn't realize when I first started telling *Michelle's Story* just how much it would help me deal with her death. I am very glad that I chose to use her story in the manner that I have. I have had several people come up to me and thank me for sharing such a personal event. In reality, I was extremely grateful to them. True to my promise that I had made to my family years earlier, I personally thanked each of them for allowing me the time and the opportunity in which to introduce her to them. I have been truly humbled over the years by the overwhelmingly positive response and the incredible impact it has had on my life. Michelle and I have certainly gone on a wonderful journey together, but for as much as that presentation has evolved, so have our travels and methods of reaching people that I never dreamed we ever could.

For a four-or-five-year period, I left the oilfield, but I continued my career in occupational safety and health by consulting in different industries, such as healthcare and agriculture. This gave me a new group of people in which to discuss the dangers of distracted driving and share my personal experiences. My state to state travels had lessened; however, the requests for speaking engagements certainly have not. I often travel within a few hours' drive from Minot to continue sharing *Michelle's Story*. But due to limited time and travel resources, I needed to find a different method to tell our family's story. It wouldn't be until I went back to work in the oil and gas industry that I would find my most creative method to date.

In July 2018, I began working for a company that had a large international presence in nearly every part of the world. As with any company in the oil extraction business, driving vehicles is, and will always be, a necessity. Often driving-related incidents occur, especially for a company that employs over 12,000 people worldwide. On my very first day there, I was introduced to our regional transportation manager, and we quickly became friends. His name was Sean, and he definitely had a strong passion for vehicle safety. He spent a significant amount of time discussing it with me. Much like every other place that I had been, he began asking me for advice about some certain driving related issues that they had been experiencing around the country and abroad. At some point in time, the topic of driving with distractions and the increasing number of vehicle accidents that they had recently experienced came up. I'm fairly confident that he was asking me because of my previous career in law enforcement, and he wanted to hear some of my many experiences and how I dealt with them. I briefly shared with him a few incidents that I had been exposed to while patrolling the streets, but I soon shared another story with him.

After telling Sean about Michelle's accident and the events surrounding it, he immediately thought of ways in which to get her story out to all our base locations, and there were many. He asked me if I would be willing to share her story.

"That's what I do," I responded. It wasn't until I began telling him about all the places I had been and the many wonderful people that I had met along the way, that he fully understood exactly what I meant.

"That's amazing," Sean said. He seemed to be in somewhat disbelief, but he continued to ask me more questions. "At some point, we need to do something together. Some project or initiative around distracted driving," he continued.

"Absolutely," I answered.

Not long after that meeting between Sean and I, one of our drivers in Texas came extremely close to losing his life in an accident that involved distractions. He was traveling on a somewhat busy and congested highway that was under construction. While traveling, his attention was diverted to his cell phone, which had been sitting on the dash. It slid off and fell to the floor by his feet. He only took his eyes off the road for mere seconds to retrieve his phone, and when he brought his focus back up to the windshield, he noticed that a semi had stopped directly in front of him. He was traveling at roughly seventy miles per hour. I couldn't imagine what must have been going through his mind at that moment. Unable to come to a complete stop, he swerved at the last second and drove the passenger side of his company truck up underneath the trailer that was attached to the semi.

Hearing this brought back so many memories of Michelle and her accident with a tractor trailer. I thought about the conversation that Sean and I had a couple months earlier. I immediately pulled out my phone and called him.

"Hey Dennis, I suppose you've already heard about the accident in Odessa?" The stress in Sean's voice was obvious.

"I have," I answered. "We were just informed in a meeting. What do you need from me?"

"I pretty much have this under control, but if you don't mind, perhaps you and I can get together on a conference call in a week or so and talk a bit more about your presentation."

I wasn't sure whether he was suggesting or asking, but either way, I knew that I needed to help him, and this company, in any way that I could.

"Not a problem," I said. "Whatever you need."

As Christmas was fast approaching, our base location in Minot experienced our own near-death vehicle incident. This time, there were three employees in a company truck, driving on an icy, minimally traveled county road, on their way out to an oilfield site. It was dark, with the only light being cast onto the roadway coming from the headlights on the pickup. Because of the heavy cloud cover, there was no additional light coming from the moon. As the driver attempted to negotiate a turn, the vehicle slid on the ice and went off the roadway. It tipped onto its side and rolled over onto its rooftop. The only thing that prevented this pickup from continuing to roll a couple hundred feet down a hillside was a conveniently positioned corner post to a cattle fence. These employees were extremely lucky to have survived this accident. This most recent event brought additional urgency on preparing and completing our planned distracted-driving training for our drivers. Over the next couple of months, Sean and I began piecing together a presentation that delved deeply into the subject of distracted driving, placing particular focus on the incidents in Odessa and Minot. The plan was for every employee in the United States, Canada, South America, and Central America to go through this training. Sean conducted the majority of the research, but as a part of the presentation, he asked me to video *Michelle's Story* so they could insert it into the training. Of course, I said yes.

In the end, we had decided that my video portion of the training would be roughly twenty minutes in length. This would be approximately half the time that it normally takes to do my presentation, so I had to find a way to get as much information as I could in a shorter timeframe than I was used to, and still make it pertinent to the company and their initiative. It was a challenge, but with Mitzie's help, I was eventually able to do it. She was the videographer and filmed me discussing *Michelle's Story* in our home with only a few takes. I didn't have the proper studio equipment or the technical knowledge necessary to professionally edit and produce a video. I was forced to continue doing individual takes until I could do it in one session without any mistakes. We spent a few hours, but we were eventually able to produce a pretty decent video. I sent it to him and eagerly awaited his response. I was fairly confident that he would like my finished product, but I needed to personally hear that from him.

"Thanks for sending your video over to me," Sean said. "I'm

currently working with some of our training folks down in Houston to get this put into the presentation."

"I assume my video will work then?" I asked.

"Oh, it's beyond what I was hoping for," he replied. "Very powerful."

With the presentation nearly finished, and the video already completed, the only thing left to do was to have the video translated for the viewers in our Central and South America bases, and then it would be time to roll this very important program out to the masses. It was determined that each location manager would deliver the presentation to their employees, and I would personally deliver it to the Minot base. Along with the presentation, the company also decided to have the severely damaged pickup from the Odessa accident transported to each base location in the United States for all the employees to see. This was a large endeavor, and I was extremely honored and proud that Michelle and I were asked to be a part of it. It was one thing for people in the United States to learn who she was, but it was entirely different for people in other countries, such as Columbia, Argentina, and Mexico, to be introduced to her.

After a few months, the distracted driving project Sean and I had put together was proving to be successful. The number of vehicle-related incidents had lowered, and managers had begun requesting that this become an annual training. Personally, my proudest moment came when employees would discuss *Michelle's Story* and related it to someone that they may have lost within their own circle. One of my safety colleagues from Mexico thanked me for sharing her story, and he explained how impactful it was when his employees discussed her accident during their safety meetings. It gave me an immense amount of pride to hear that, but more than anything, I was happy to spark conversation around the dangers of driving with distractions. We were certainly achieving that.

As successful as this latest venture had been, my journey with

Michelle continued to move forward, and we continued meeting incredibly wonderful people all over. I continued speaking at other events around the state, both in the occupational setting and in public forums. Word had gotten around about this guy from Minot, North Dakota who had a tragic story about distracted driving and the devastating effects it can have on a family. Many people continued to request it. As long as there are people that are willing to open their minds and hearts and give me an hour of their precious time, I will continue to share her story.

———

GRIEF AND DEPRESSION ARE TWO UGLY MONSTERS THAT often go hand in hand with each other. Both are equally dangerous and once they get you secured in their grasp, escaping their hold becomes extremely difficult—if not impossible—without some help. If I've learned anything since my sister's car accident, it's that dealing with the death of a loved one is an emotional rollercoaster ride, with many ups and downs, twists and turns. Mostly you just want it to come to an end. You want the hurt and uncertainty to stop. You want the healing to begin.

I've had the unfortunate opportunity to watch these monsters destroy my mother's life and have learned several years later how they quietly impacted my father. I felt my brother's grief echo through the phone as we talked, and I saw the emotional toll it took on Penny by the stress that was often visibly displayed on her face. I watched our sister, Denise, completely melt down after Michelle's death, only to watch her later deal with the devastating loss of a child herself. Through it all, I was unable to do anything for each of them. I thought that I was being strong, being that rock that each of them had grown to depend on. But in reality, I was hurting just as much. I simply refused to talk about it. Some of my family members couldn't escape those monsters, while others, such as Dad and I, never even knew they were there.

When our mother was spending her final days in the hospital in Coudersport, Pennsylvania, Penny, Mike and Denise left many of the decisions up to me. At least that's what the physicians told me when Mitzie and I arrived that chilly winter evening. I was honored that they all felt comfortable enough and had the trust in me to make the right decisions. I mostly hoped that I wouldn't let them down. After Mom had passed away, Denise told me that she considered me her hero. Little did she know that she, Penny, and Mike were all my heroes. There were times in my life when I needed each one of them, Michelle included, and they were all there for me.

We were never a family that said "I love you," to each other while growing up, but after Michelle's death, we all became closer. When our parents both died, we became a tight, cohesive unit with an unbreakable bond. We've always been different bunch, but I couldn't think of any other people that I would want to call my siblings, and I love each one of them. They have each helped me fight off the grief and depression over the years, and sharing Michelle's story has helped me bring peace and acceptance to my life.

———

THE WORDS TO *MICHELLE'S STORY* CAN OFTEN BE SEEN during my presentations as they roll quietly out of the corners of my eyes and make their way down my cheeks, before eventually being swiped away with the palm of my hand, tucking her memory safely away in my heart.

It's been a great journey so far, Michelle, but our work has only just begun. There are still people who want to meet you.

The sun makes its way up into the vast Texas sky. It pushes the darkness of night away and brings with it new opportunities and immense possibilities. Turning away from my hotel window, I sat my nearly empty cardboard cup down on a small wooden table that was tucked tightly into the corner. I reached for my briefcase that had been quietly waiting in a leather office chair beside the bed. I opened the door, lowered my head and smiled, quietly uttering to myself, "Let's go make some new friends Michelle."

EPILOGUE

I didn't know what to expect when I decided to take on this monumental challenge of writing a book. In fact, I never thought that I would ever write a book, and I really didn't write this one. This story has been writing itself since the summer of 2005, when Dean was first diagnosed with cancer. When I finally decided it was time to take Michelle's story to the next level, I knew that I wouldn't be able to do it without the help of my brother and sisters. I didn't know how they would react to me putting our family's history, both good and bad, out there for the world to read for themselves. To my surprise, they were more than accepting, even though they all knew that they would have to dig deep into their own personal libraries and pull out some painful memories. To their credit, each one of them was up to the challenge.

Writing this book was both an incredible and emotional journey that forced me and my family to relive difficult moments surrounding the sudden loss of our sister, Michelle. I spent a great deal of time talking with each of my family members about the feelings that they experienced after Michelle's death. I described, as best as I could, how everyone was immediately affected by her death, but I wanted them to try to explain it in their own words. Although their responses differed from one another, they each shared remarkable stories that clearly illustrates the raw emotions that they felt upon learning about her car accident and how it has affected them in the years since. As I read through their letters, I could hear their obvious sadness, a bit of anger, and some very fond memories that they happily shared. It was important for me to include them in this book because there was so much more to this tragedy than just Michelle dying. Her death had a tremendous impact on so many lives, certainly much more than I described in this book. Here are some of their stories.

"On October 6, 2005, we lost, not only our baby sister, but also our mother, because she was never the same after that. A piece of her died that fateful day. In the time span of an hour, maybe less, we buried a future brother-in-law, left the cemetery, went searching for Michelle, talked to numerous people, including the Highway Patrol, saw the gentleman that was driving the 18-Wheeler that ended our sister's life, and then had to begin making arrangements to bury our sister.

Mad?? No, I'm not mad per say. I am angry that a tropical storm by the name of "Tammy" was sitting just off the coast of Wilmington giving us a good dose of rain that was literally coming down every way imaginable, to the tune of 1 foot by the time we left there a day later. I'm angry that we didn't INSIST that Michelle just go back to Dean's parent's house with us and pick her car up from Andrews Mortuary later. I'm angry because she left so many people behind to deal with this, her siblings and parents, not to mention her 3 sons.

So, how has it affected me??? Have you ever pulled up on the scene of an accident, knowing full well that it was YOUR FAMILY MEMBER?? I still have my days, like the day I closed my eyes and had to once again relive EVERY moment of that day for my brother's book. All because of a storm and distracted driving !!"

Penny Pettengill (Sister)

"Growing up, I was close to Michelle. We were very close in our teen years. She was not only my cousin, but like a sister I never had. She would spend many nights with me and we would spend whole weekends playing Monopoly, except when we were sleeping. In my adult life, I spent numerous hours on the phone with Michelle, talking about our kids, our parents, and our everyday lives. I will never forget the last time I spoke with her. It was the day before her accident. She had called me to talk about Dean's funeral. She told me that she would call me later the next day. Never did I dream it would be the last time I would speak to her. The next day I got a call from Denise telling me Michelle had died. That phone call rocked me to the core. I was in such disbelief. Since then I know Michelle's spirit has been around to visit me. About a year after she passed, I was vacuuming my floors, and after I was finished, I found a piece of paper on my dining room floor with her phone number on it, that she had given me years earlier. There isn't a day that goes by that I do not miss her. She will be forever missed and loved!"

— Ronda Reynolds (Cousin)

"When recalling the day of Michelle's accident, it was a normal day for me, just relaxing in my chair after work, and watching tv when Mitzie called to say that Michelle was in a car accident after leaving

Dean's funeral. I thought it was just a minor fender bender, so I wasn't terribly alarmed, and figured I would be getting a call from Michelle, telling me all about it. After some time had passed, another call came in from Mitzie, except this time she was crying, and I knew something wasn't right. My heart sank. At that moment, I found out Michelle hadn't survived the accident, and Mitzie kept saying, "She's gone, she's gone." I just froze. I don't remember hanging up or saying goodbye to Mitzie. I was just thinking, "Oh no, this isn't happening. Not now, not ever!" All I could do was stare out the window, in shock, for what seemed like an eternity before I gathered my thoughts, and went to Carrie, my wife, and gave her a hug and said, "Michelle's gone."

My thoughts then went to my parents and siblings, and thinking, "How are we going to get through this tragedy?" I have always carried some guilt by not being down there for her during her time of need, then maybe she would still be with us. Just maybe. This keeps me up at nights wondering, what if?

Beyond that, the next few days were a blur until we all gathered at our parents' home, in Ohio, to prepare for her funeral service and to say goodbye. A piece of me died along with her, and life won't ever be the same, but I try and move past it with some humor because if I can make others laugh and smile, that helps me heal a little bit more.

I am constantly recalling stories of Michelle that make me smile, or wonder what she was thinking. One time, we had a little red wagon, so my brother and I decided it would be fun to push her down a big cement ramp by the park in Mannington, West Virginia, where we lived. So, we did, and she crashed at the bottom, and we got spanked by our dad. Poor Michelle was always our test subject growing up. We just thought, "If she can survive, we can to." There was another time my brother and I took it upon ourselves to teach Michelle how to ride her bike, and there again, involved a hill. We gave her a push and, down the hill she went, pretty fast, but to our surprise, she didn't crash. One more story I often recall is when Michelle was around ten years old. We lived in Shinglehouse, Pennsylvania. Our parents were going somewhere, and she wanted to go with them, but she had to stay with a sitter. This didn't sit well with her, so she punched the living room window, shattering it, and she had to be taken to the hospital to receive several stitches.

To say the least, Michelle kept things interesting. She's always been a free spirit, and that's what made her unique. She held on to that until she left us. Her niece, my daughter, who was born years after Michelle was gone, and who is also her namesake, Neva Michelle, is carrying on her Aunt Michelle's free-spirited nature. I think this child came into our lives to remind us who Michelle was and to carry on her legacy. She's doing a great job! Michelle would have been so proud.

So, to conclude, I miss you every day Michelle, and thanks for the memories. You will never be forgotten!

— MIKE SNODGRASS (BROTHER)

"I will never forget the few days leading up to my sister Michelle's tragic death. I got a phone call as soon as I got into work that early morning from my Michelle and she was crying hysterically. I was in Ohio and she was in North Carolina. I had to calm her down enough to understand what she was trying to tell me. When she did finally calm down a bit, she told me that she was woke up by her fiancé, Dean Manning, and that he had been experiencing some bleeding, that was related to his cancer treatments. Dean had been diagnosed with non-Hodgkin's lymphoma a few months earlier and had been in the hospital the majority of that time. Michelle was staying in the hospital with him and going to work every day, from there. Well, this particular morning he was bleeding very badly. He woke Michelle up and said he felt wet and she turned on the light. At this point, she became alarmed and scared. She called for the nurses and they had her leave the room. This was when she called me about five O'clock in the morning crying. Dean passed away that evening. The bleeding was a result of a blood infection from the chemotherapy he was taking.

A few days later, Dean's funeral was held and Michelle was heartbroken. At this time in North Carolina, a terrible tropical storm was passing through, and it was bad. After leaving the funeral home, all of the guests proceeded to the cemetery. I was unable to be there for Michelle because I could not leave Ohio due to a previous appointment that I could not reschedule. Shortly after Dean's funeral, Michelle was killed because her car hydroplaned in the massive downpour of this tropical storm. I was at work that evening when I got a phone call from my mother. I learned that she had been on the phone with Michelle and heard her scream "Oh my God"! The phone went dead after that and mom was unable to get Michelle back on the phone. She then called me and was so worried, but I told her that Michelle was fine and that she was just stressed and that her phone had probably needed charged. Little did I know that I was very, very wrong. After work, I went to my mom and dad's house. My son bubby, Paul, was there sitting on the couch. I was only there a few minutes when mom got the phone call from my brother in law, Ed Pettengill. He had told her that Michelle was with the angels and Dean now. From my end I heard her say, "She's gone?" I didn't believe it for a few minutes and looked over at my son. He had his head hanging over the end of the couch. He already knew what my mind was refusing to believe. My dad walked over and told me that we all have to stick together and stay calm. He was shaking very badly, and this was when I knew that Michelle had been killed. I kept saying "no" and shaking my head and then, I ran out of the apartment crying.

I lost a piece of my heart that day, and my life has never been the same since. Michelle was my best friend and a second mother to *my children, who were very heartbroken by this news. I miss her and think about her often. I want to talk to her again and let her know that she is a grandmother now, but that's going to have to wait.*

This is why I never talk on the phone while I am driving."

— DENISE SNODGRASS CUSTER (SISTER)

OF COURSE, MY LIFE, AND THIS BOOK, WOULDN'T BE complete without the strength and loving support that I've received for so many years from my beautiful partner, Mitzie. I'm not sure I would have been able to handle so much loss without having her beside me to help me through it all. Here are her words.

Dennis,

I have known you and your family for over 20 years and consider them my own, and love them with all my heart. You and I have been together through all of the hardships and tragedies you have written about in your book, and I have never regretted any of it. You are my best friend and soulmate. I cannot think of living my life without you in it. Everything I do or contemplate doing, I always think of you first. You are a wonderful father, a SUPER grandpa, and the best friend I could ever ask for. I was very lucky that day some 24 years ago when you walked into the reserve center and said hi. Who would have known that all these years later we would have 5 terrific kids and be blessed with 10 of the best grandchildren? Never in all the time we have been together have you disappointed me. You have taken care of our entire family through all the tough times. I think sometimes you are the rock we all lean on too much, and sometimes you need a rock also. I want you to know that I will forever be your rock. I am grateful that you came into my life and what a wonderful life it has been so far. Even in my lowest moments you can make me smile and will do whatever you have to, to make me laugh. I will love you forever.

    ~Mitzie

LETTER TO THE READER

It has been a true honor to have been able to write this book. Although nearly everyone is exposed to some form of distracted driving in their lifetime, I feel the subject doesn't seem to garner enough attention until something tragic happens. It is my personal opinion that more consideration seems to be given to drunk driving, rather than distracted driving; however, both are equally as dangerous. Both claim lives. Each leave families shattered. No matter how advanced vehicles become, and no matter how many visual distractions the automakers build into each one, it is still up to the individual drivers to manage the various distractions that they are exposed to and make every effort possible to do the right thing in order to keep themselves, and other motorists on the highways, safe during their respective travels.

One question that often comes up when I speak to people is, "What about hands-free while driving?" The only thing that this accomplishes is it frees up the driver's hands. Their eyes may stay on the road ahead of them, but their mind's eye is usually wherever the other half of that conversation is, especially if the conversation isn't going well.

Often times, driving with distractions is a conscious decision of the driver. So many times, drivers will reach down and pick up their cellphones without likely giving it much thought. Since the time that I first began sharing Michelle's story, it has been my hope that if we were able to accomplish anything, it would be that her story would bring some much-needed thought and discussion to this very important topic. I've said several times before I never wanted to tell this story, but it's a story that needed to be told.

I've also learned so many things since Michelle's unfortunate passing. Things that I never thought I would ever learn or even gave a second thought to. I learned things about myself, my family, and the process associated with grief, but mostly, I learned a few things about death itself.

I learned that death plays no favorites and doesn't discriminate. Death doesn't care how old you are, or how successful you may have become throughout your life. It doesn't care if you're rich or poor, or comfortable or not. Death doesn't care about a person's employment history, political status, or religious preference. None of these have any bearing on death.

It makes no difference whether you think about death, whether or not you accept it, or even if you fear it. No, death simply doesn't care. In the end, death will claim everyone. We can presumably hold death off for a while, depending on how we choose to live our lives and with some of the decisions we make, but I firmly believe that when our time comes, death will eagerly come for us all.

One last thing that I learned through the process of writing this book is, death doesn't care how you're feeling or where you've been in your life, even if you just left your fiancée's funeral, so my advice to everyone is, cherish your family and loved ones. Tell them you love them every day, because in the end, we don't know how long they'll be with us.

PHOTOS

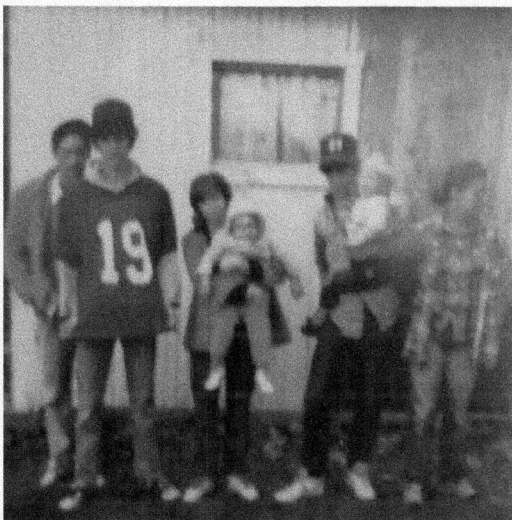

The Cabin in Ohio: (Left to Right) Dad, Dennis, Michelle, Mike & Mom, two cousins

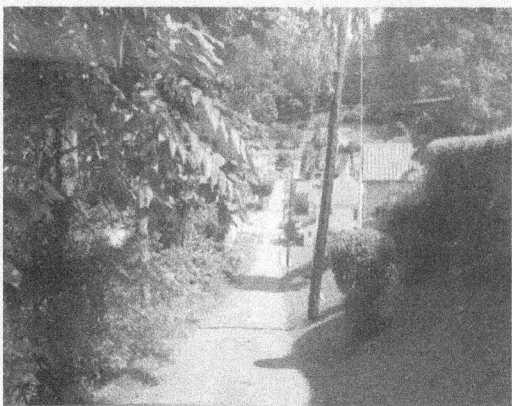

Farmington, WV: Looking down the hill.

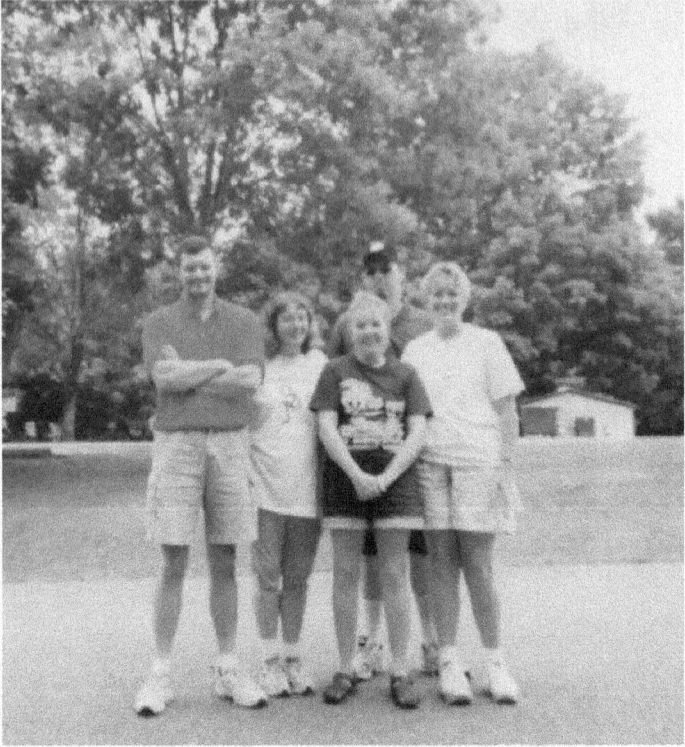

Wolf Run, Ohio: (Left to Right) Dennis, Michelle, Mike, Denise, Penny

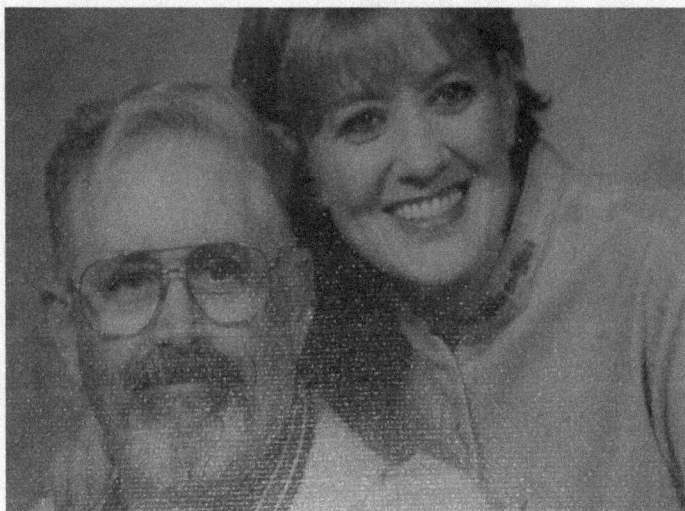

Penny and Ed

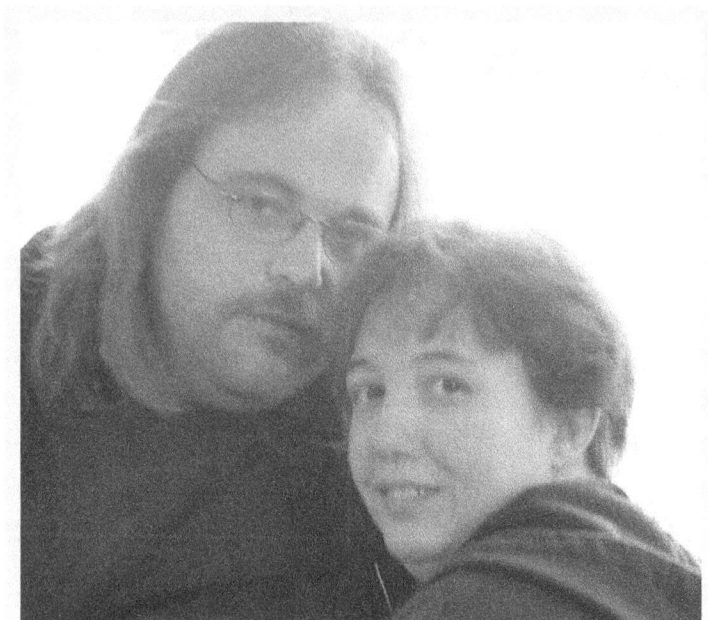

Michelle and Dean

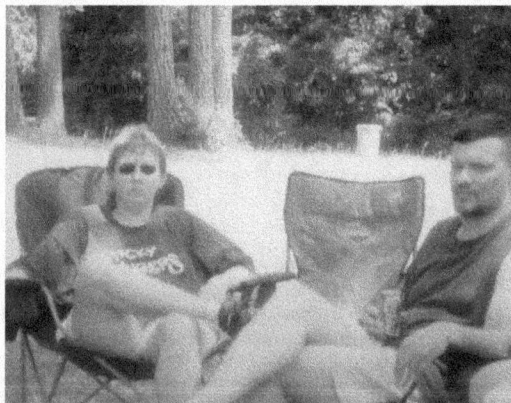

Michelle and Dennis at Fort Fisher

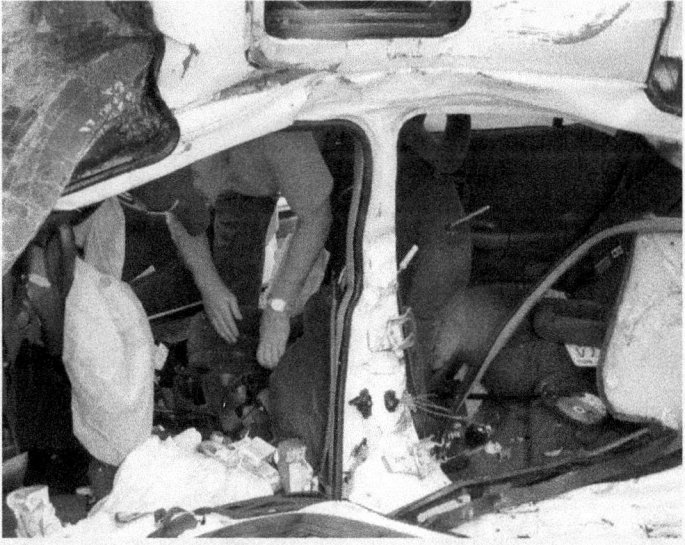
Michelle's Car after the accident.

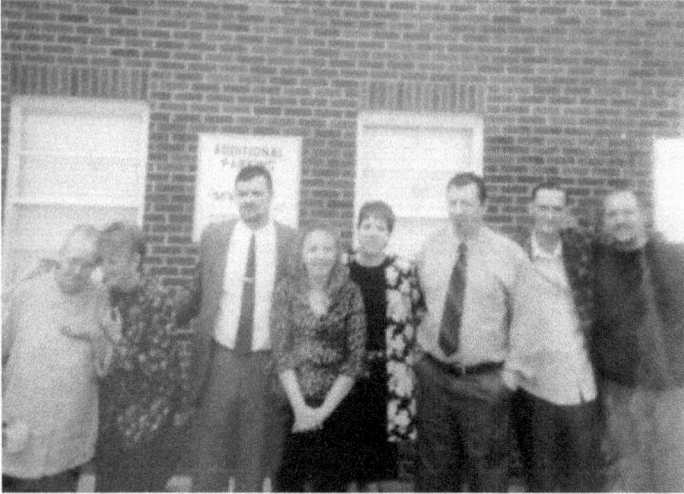

Michelle's Funeral: (Left to Right) Mom, Penny, Dennis, Denise, Sherry, Mike, Dad, and Chris

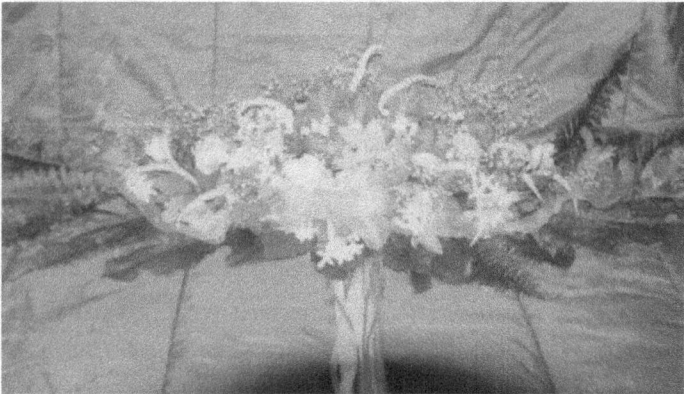

Floral Spray made for Michelle's funeral.

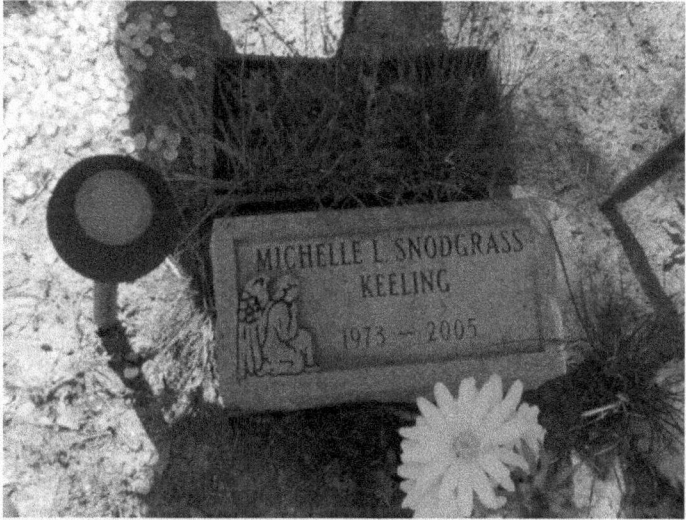

Michelle's Stone

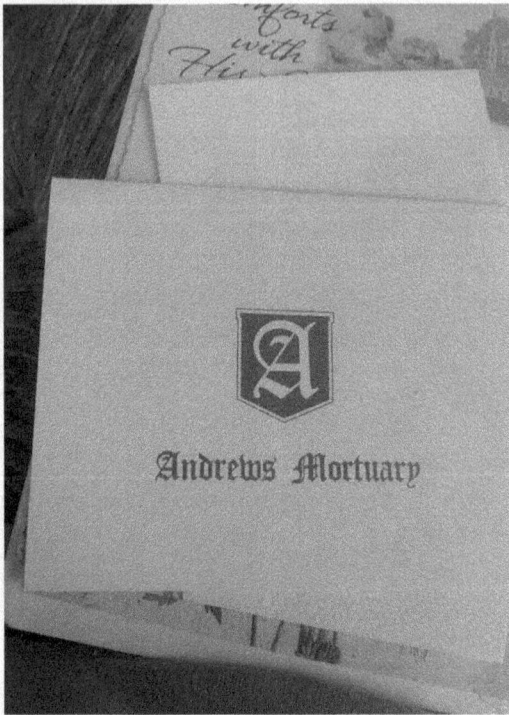

Card received by Dean from Andrew's Mortuary

Dear Penny,
I am sorry we have been unable to connect by phone. I want to extend my deepest sympathy to you and your family over the death of your sister, Michele. I have enclosed my card to let you know that you can call if you need any bereavement support. Peace and Grace to you,

Speaks for itself.

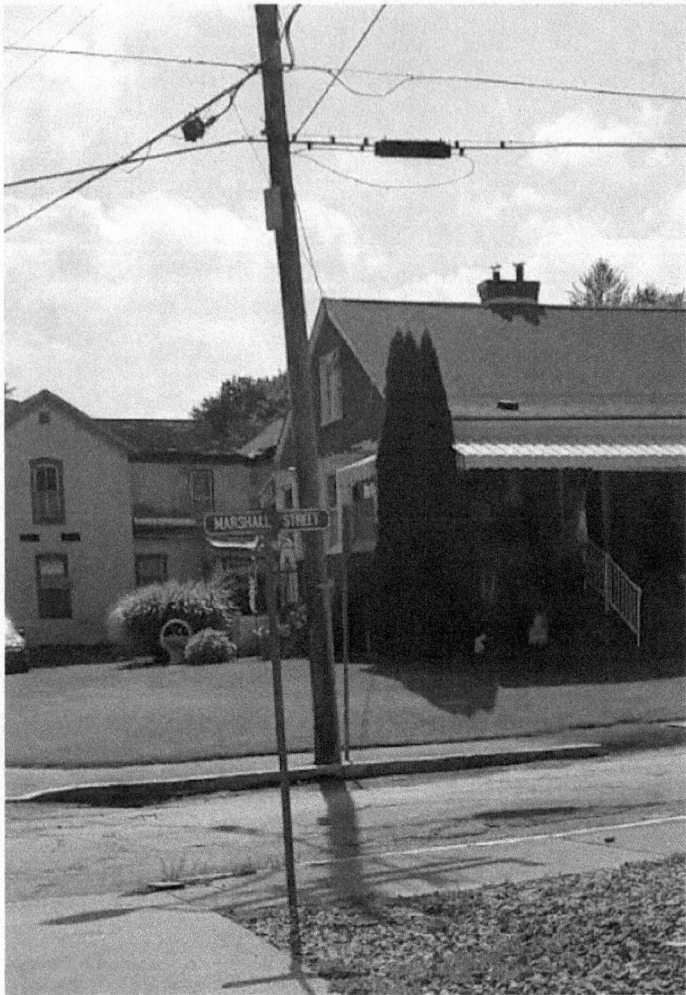

Marshall Street, Mannington, WV

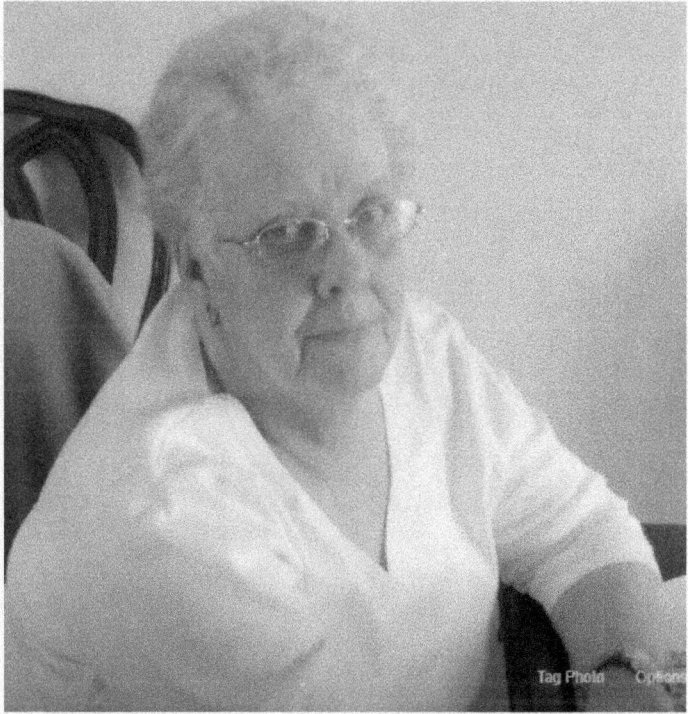

Mom

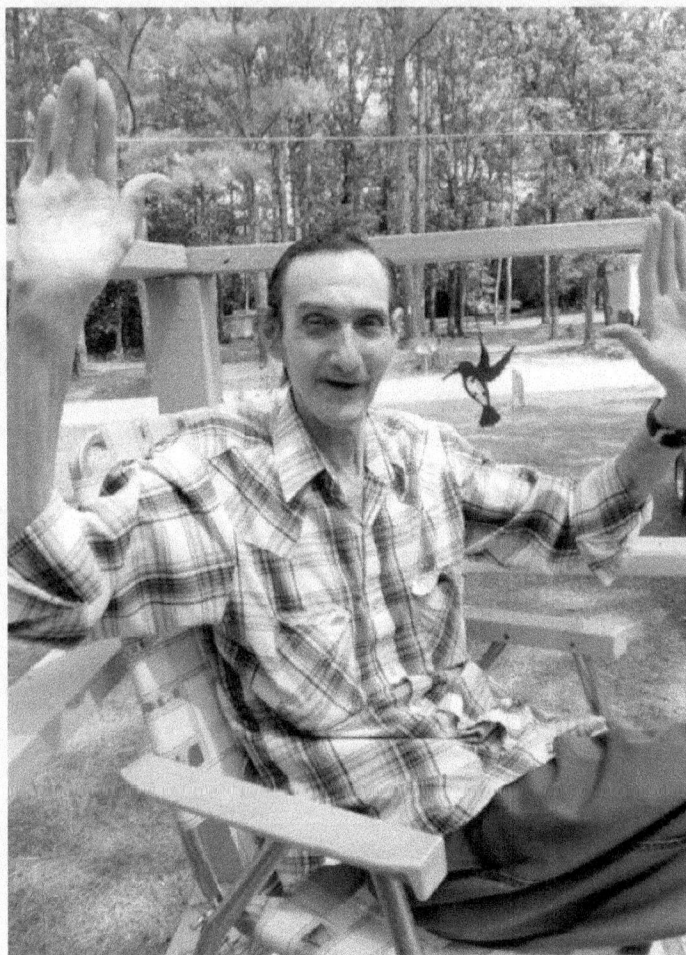

Dad: A year before he passed away.

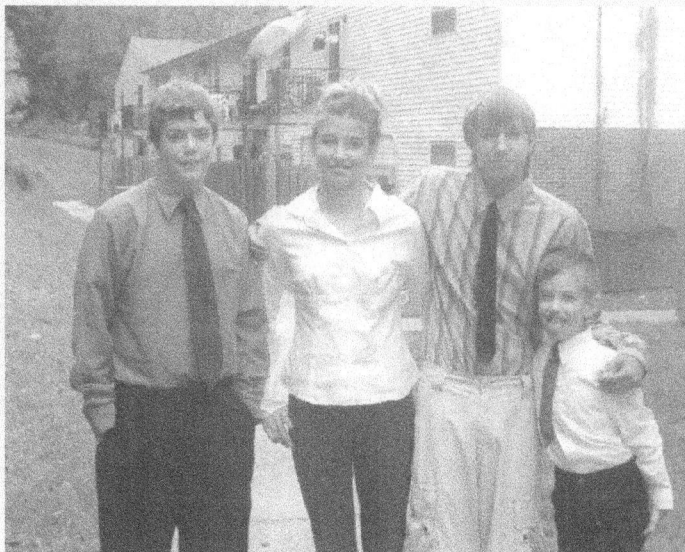

(Left to Right) Jared, Amanda, Shawn, and Nicky

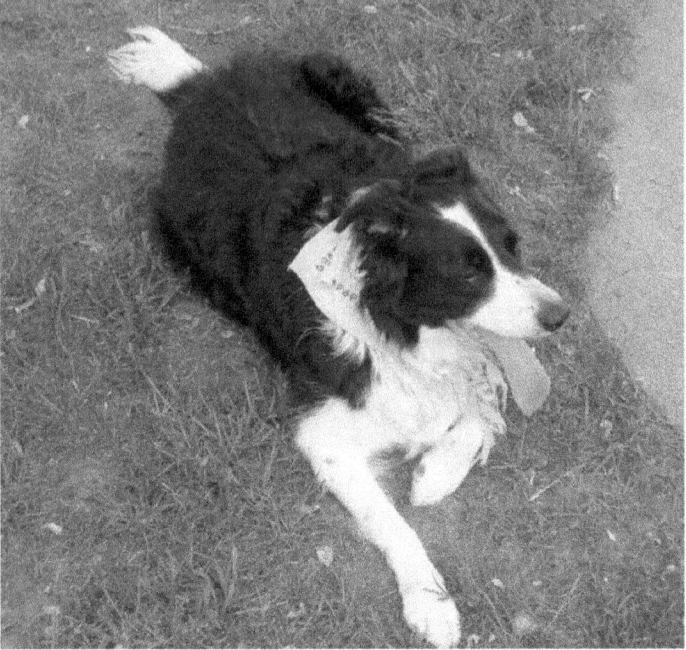
Skeeter "Pete"

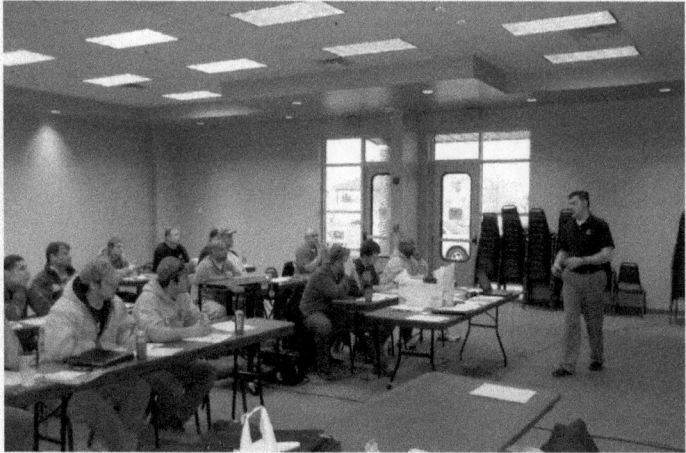

Greeley, Colorado: Dennis delivering "Michelle's Story"

ACKNOWLEDGMENTS

I want to thank some very special people who have enriched my life and helped make this world a much better place to live.

Thank you Mom, Dad, Michelle, Penny, Mike, Denise, Chris, and Sherry for all your support and encouragement. A very special thank you to Mitzie, Amanda, Shawn, Zack, Jared, and Nick for your unconditional love.

And, thank you Pastor Wayne for helping my parents find hope and comfort in their lives.

I love all of you!

ABOUT THE AUTHOR

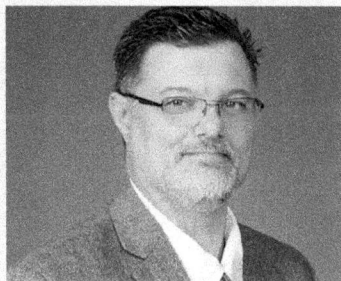

Dennis is a safety professional in the brutal oilfields of North Dakota, former Police Chief, and a Marine Corps veteran. However, the titles he cherishes most are that of father and grandfather. Through training, mentoring, and consulting, Dennis has dedicated his life to helping others that may not have the ability to help themselves. He never envisioned himself as an author, but after spending nearly a decade sharing his very personal and impactful story about his sister's untimely death, Dennis finally decided to put those powerful words on paper and wrote his first book, *"Passing Through the Storm."*

f facebook.com/dennis.snodgrass.3551
🐦 twitter.com/1005publishing